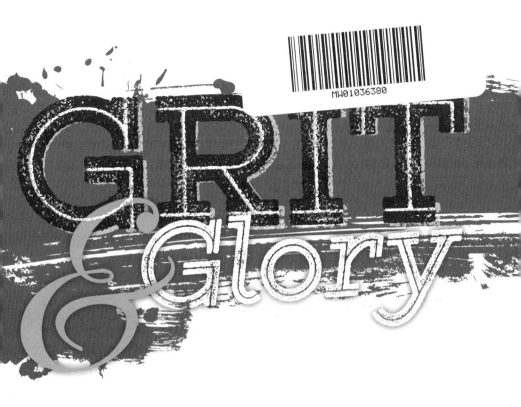

GRIT
& Glory

KAISER
JOHNSON

**Our
Sunday
Visitor**

www.osv.com
Our Sunday Visitor Publishing Division
Our Sunday Visitor, Inc.
Huntington, Indiana 46750

Our Sunday Visitor Publishing Division
Our Sunday Visitor, Inc.
200 Noll Plaza
Huntington, IN 46750
1-800-348-2440

ISBN: 978-1-68192-232-4 (Inventory No. T1933)
eISBN: 978-1-68192-233-1
LCCN: 2017964304

Cover design: Tyler Ottinger
Interior design: Lindsey Riesen
Photography: Mark Lewandowski

PRINTED IN THE UNITED STATES OF AMERICA

CONTENTS

INTRODUCTION

"Work therefore and pray, says our Lord, that you enter not into temptation."
—Thomas à Kempis, *The Imitation of Christ*

Catholics believe that we're truly a union of body and spirit, but in practice many unbelievers live that out better than we do.

I'm talking about those who have an integrated spiritual and physical life. In my own Los Angeles area that includes yoga-obsessed people, dedicated "CrossFitters" (those in the CrossFit program), disciples of martial arts, and "surfing gurus." Their devotion to their physical activity or sport informs their faith practice, or at least their philosophy of life, and vice versa.

They practice what they preach… even if I can't fully agree with their preaching.

Yoga moms demonstrate patience and endurance in their training, and aspire to it in their personal lives. CrossFitters seek out dedication and devotion to what they at least see as "heroic" feats, both in and out of the CrossFit "box" (translation: gym). Surfers learn (as Catholic philosopher and professor Dr. Peter Kreeft points out) detachment and trust in something bigger than themselves (the wave and the ocean).

But what about us?

We Catholics extol the importance of virtue, of fortitude, of detachment, of trust, of patience, of suffering… and yet, many of us think of fitness as vanity, or sports as a spectator pastime. When we do that, we miss the great opportunity God gives us to practice our values in our bodies on a daily basis, and in doing so, truly influencing how we behave and interact with the world throughout our lives.

As Saint Paul says: "I do not run aimlessly, I do not box as one beating the air; but I pommel my body and subdue it, lest after preaching to others I myself should be disqualified" (1 Cor 9:26–27). Although it would certainly be a stretch to say he's talking about fitness training here, he's undeniably talking about the integral connection between how he treats and challenges his body and how he works out his salvation.

Yes, there are ways to practice discipline and mortification like fasting, cold showers, regular devotions, and so on. Why ignore or run away from discipline and sacrifice that directly affect our health and physical well-being, that tend to our "temples of the Holy Spirit"? I think if we're honest, the real answer is that we fear making a commitment to what we're sure will be protracted difficulty and suffering. Many of us then try to use our faith to justify this fear, rather than drawing on our faith to do something good for our bodies... and, in fact, our souls!

It's true there are potential pitfalls to fitness, but they're similar to pitfalls that exist in the seeking of any beneficial practice. Throughout our lives as Catholics, we generally find our greatest temptations not in things totally contrary to our faith, but more in misusing, or over- or underemphasizing, a great good. So just as we find the importance of both feasting and fasting, public and private prayer, work and rest, if we approach fitness properly, we'll gain great discipline and virtue, without falling into obsessiveness, vanity, or the like.

Now, what if you love fitness but find living a spiritual life difficult, or feel more "spiritual than religious," or just "can't be bothered"? A second ago I mentioned that I think "if we're honest" we understand our real hesitancy to working out. I also think that "if we're honest," we know deep in our hearts that if we have a daily practice for our bodies, but not our souls, we're only half living. We might say we're "doing just fine" the way we are, but one of the lessons we know from fitness is that "doing just fine" doesn't cut it.

If we want to compete, to grow stronger, to lift more, to be leaner, we don't accept "doing just fine" from ourselves. A favorite motivational sports quote of mine is, "We were not created for an easy life, but for great things, for goodness." These words might have been spoken by John Wooden or Vince Lombardi... but they weren't. They were spoken by Pope Benedict XVI, and, okay, it's not technically a sports quote, but it works! (The full quote, if you're interested, goes, "The ways of the Lord are not easy, but we were not created for an easy life, but for great things, for goodness.") You're made for great things, not to be "just fine." You're made for a fully integrated life, one in which your body and soul work together. You're made to live out goodness, dedication, and health in every aspect of your existence. You're made to live the practice of faith: praying when prayer seems difficult or hopeless or useless, knowing and doing the right thing when it feels impossible, finding God and good in suffering (whether we choose the suffering or it happens to us against our will). All these have the power to make us an integrated person and provide a fully satisfying life, one spent living the greatness for which God created us.

For living out goodness, dedication, and health in every aspect of your existence. For living out the practice of faith: praying when prayer seems difficult or hopeless or useless; knowing and doing the right thing when it feels impossible; finding God and good in suffering (whether we choose the suffering or it happens to us against our will). All these have the power to make us an integrated person and provide a fully satisfying life, one spent living the greatness for which God created us.

That's the aim of this book: to lay out the central principles for a healthy physical life, as well as the principles for a healthy spiritual life ... which coincidentally are the same. I'll go through the building blocks of losing weight, improving performance, getting stronger and leaner, as well as the building blocks of detachment, improving virtue, and becoming more disciplined in spiritual growth. These principles apply both to men and women, young and old, and the physical fitness plans and spiritual fitness plans are adaptable to different goals and starting places.

A quick background on me, with full disclosure: Everything I have to offer is what I've learned and applied in my own life. I don't have a formal education in either faith or fitness. However, I've very effectively worked in both worlds. I came back to my Catholic faith in college when a friend began asking me challenging questions about my nominal faith. I dove into studying the Church, the saints, and why Catholics believe what they believe.

The result? I found myself returning to where I know I belong.

Since then I've written and produced a catechetical web series (*Young Catholic Minute*) that was picked up and remade by EWTN. I've hosted multiple other Catholic series, now lead the Hollywood Chesterton Society, and speak professionally on G. K. Chesterton. In the fitness world, I've worked as a personal trainer, and compete in obstacle racing at an elite level, which keeps me focused on the cutting edge of training in strength, speed, and endurance, as well as nutrition and performance. In short, faith and fitness occupy nearly every moment of my life in one capacity or another, and that combination gives me a useful perspective on the matter.

Secular friends have often asked me how I live with discipline and integrity in my personal life, which they see as an impossible or burdensome task. Catholic friends have often asked how I live with discipline and integrity in my physical life, which they see as an impossible or burdensome task. But one thing we learn from the Incarnation is that for all of us life should be lived as an integrated whole, not two separate parts. Exercise and fitness are a place to begin for some, and prayer and faith are a starting line for others. Together, they can radically change the lives of Catholics and non-Catholics alike. With that in mind, let's get started.

PART 1
The Concepts

CHAPTER ONE
The Desire to Grow and Change

"You, therefore, must be perfect, as your heavenly Father is perfect."
— Matthew 5:48

The single, most essential positive influence in my life boils down to one thing: every day, every minute, every second, I want to be growing, learning, and changing for the better. I do it badly most of the time, but that's my desire, and I work to live in accord with it. Having the desire to be perfect, and the humble willingness to be obedient to that process, is the starting place. It's the only way we make genuine progress.

Mark tells us when Jesus visited his hometown of Nazareth after beginning his public ministry, most everyone there couldn't understand how "the carpenter, the son of Mary" could suddenly do mighty works and teach with such authority. Because of this unbelief, this lack of cooperation with grace, Jesus, "could do no mighty work there, except that he laid his hands upon a few sick people and healed them" (Mk 6:5.) While God's power and grace are unlimited, if we won't let them in, he won't force them on us. Whereas if we do open ourselves up to grace, we can move mountains (see Mt 17:20)! The same holds true for us in *every* aspect of our lives.

Productivity expert Brian Tracy says that most of us live on "Someday Isle," where we spend our time saying "someday I'll …" and fill in the blank. We swap excuses and think about our good intentions instead of taking meaningful action to grow and change. And to borrow at least a close paraphrase attributed to Saint Bernard of Clairvaux, "the road to hell is paved with good intentions."

So the desire to grow and change — to be "perfect" — must be quickly followed with action, with doing, or it will quickly become cemented as a *desire* daydreamed about rather than a *habit* lived out. In this book, you'll receive a lot of information, hopefully some inspiration, and a game plan for the next 9 days, 21 days, 40 days, and 90 days. But unless you want to make these a part of your life, unless you really want to and will make more prayer, reflection, and care for your body a part of your life, they won't be.

Maybe you're starting at a place where you say: "My prayer life is on point! I just need to get myself in the gym." Or maybe the reverse is true: "My gym life is on point! I just need to get myself to church" Then again, maybe you think you've got everything — or nothing — figured out. The truth is no matter where you're at in your spiritual life, and no matter where you're at in your life of fitness, you have plenty of room to grow.

Remember, every day from today to the last breath you take is an opportunity for growth, and to become closer to God and to all he truly desires to give you. As Pope Saint John Paul II said, "Become who you are." Who you really are, who you are at your core, is a fully integrated part of humanity, body and soul, in complete union and harmony. The real you fully expressed is someone who inspires those around you, serves as an example for those who desire good, and is a stumbling block to those who don't.

At the risk of over-quoting people smarter than I am, Saint Irenaeus said, "The glory of God is man fully alive." God created us in his image. Yes, it's been distorted by sin, but every one of us has the capacity to live out God's glory more fully every day for the rest of our lives. Too often we say to ourselves, "I'm good where I'm at." So here's my question: are you in heaven? Because if you're not, then you're not good where you're at.

I've heard people point out that they're done with school and conclude that they no longer need to learn, say that their doctor said their cholesterol is fine, so they don't need to lose weight, and that, after all, they already know how not to kill anyone or steal, so why go to church? The problem with all of these is that we're setting false standards for ourselves... and really low ones at that. Jesus doesn't call us to be better than the worst we can imagine, or to be better than the bare minimum. Remember, he says, "Be perfect, therefore, as your heavenly Father is perfect." Too often we compare ourselves to the wrong standard: the floor below us instead of the sky Christ offers us. The Christ who told us to "be perfect."

Making progress toward perfection will be a painful process ... one we generally won't complete before heaven. As Saint Francis de Sales teaches, on this side of eternity, there's only progress and not perfection. Even Jesus, who is perfection itself, suffered intensely. And Mary, who also wasn't spiritually disfigured by sin like the rest of us, still experienced her seven sorrows, which probably would have done in the rest of us. All the saints have suffered. As Jesus tells us, "If any man would come after me, let him deny himself and take up his cross daily and follow me" (Lk 9:23). The way to perfection isn't easy, but it *is* worth it.

When Revelation speaks of heaven, it warns us, "nothing unclean shall enter it" (21:27). Heaven is on the line, so let's live like it. Every time I'm tempted to say, "I'm too busy to pray," or "No one will notice this sin," or "What does it matter what I do with my body?" I let the great gift God desires to give me slip through my fingers, rather than treasuring it with every ounce of my being.

Now, this is a book on faith and fitness. You might think that I overstate the importance of fitness … or that I overstate the importance of faith. The fact is even using the words "body" and "soul" almost draws a false distinction. Until we take our dying breath there's no separating them. (And then only until the end of time and the resurrection of the body.) We're called to a fully integrated life, and that integration means living with integrity. So let's prepare ourselves to offer our prayers, works, joys, and sufferings... *all* of ourselves to God. That's the starting point, and the only way we have the potential to change.

Don't settle for anything less!

CHAPTER TWO
Suffering

"If we only knew the precious treasure hidden in infirmities, we would receive them with the same joy with which we receive the greatest benefits, and we would bear them without ever complaining or showing signs of weariness."
— Saint Vincent de Paul

Catholics often have a strange relationship with suffering — one that vacillates between near masochism in penitence or asceticism on one hand, and the refusal to practice self-discipline and restraint in actual practical matters like diet and exercise on the other. I've known Catholics who indiscriminately heap on devotions, but rationalize having a dinner consisting of cake and ice cream because "the physical is less important than the spiritual." They run away from effort and physical activity and say, "God doesn't care how I look."

The other side of the coin is the people who "can't" find an hour on Sundays to make it to Mass, but easily find an hour daily to exercise. They fit in work, play, and workouts without missing a beat, but with all that are "too busy" to give God any time.

The reality is that these people are actually doing the same thing most humans are best at: serving ourselves. When Saint Irenaeus said, "The glory of God is man fully alive," he didn't say, "the glory of God is man ignoring the body and trying to make up for it by doing extra soul work." He also didn't say, "The glory of God is man with a killer bod." I'll say it again: to be truly Catholic, we don't separate our body and soul… but live as an integrated whole, as the embodied spirits God created us to be.

In our lives, God allows us sufficient suffering to perfect us. However, we need to accept that suffering, not run away from it and pick out a different kind of suffering we're okay with or, worse, are really excited to wallow in.

We'll all experience heartbreak and tragedy that tries our souls along the way. But more often we'll experience the natural stress to our hearts and minds that trying to live a basic functional life brings. We get to offer all of that, both the big and small, both the life changing and the base line, to God. If I spend an hour in adoration, but spend an hour cursing LA drivers and stress-eating the candy bar I picked up at the gas station, what have I gained? If I go to church daily, but daily refuse to take care of my body, the temple of the Holy Spirit that God has entrusted to me, I'm missing the point.

God has given us bodies that need tending, that respond to exercise, that serve us better the more we put them into service. He's also allowed that process to provide a fair amount of suffering. Why avoid that? God is giving you the opportunity to tend to the temple. It won't be easy, but it will be worth doing.

Again, on the flip side, if you're someone who says, "the gym is my church," or "hiking is how I'm with God," or "Sundays are for football or sleeping in," you're deceiving yourself. You can certainly offer the suffering of an extra set to God. You can certainly pray and feel close to God surrounded by his magnificent creation. You can certainly use playing a sport to love your neighbor and your enemy (you know, maybe your teammate and your opponent?) all at once. But if that takes you away from offering God the worship he asks of you, you're missing the point. If you glorify the body to the detriment of your soul, you set up an opposition that shouldn't exist, and you become less human, less fully alive, and less of who you actually are. At times, attending Mass, praying, or going to confession can be far from easy. But they are always good, maybe especially when they involve a kind of suffering. They give us an opportunity to tend the temple.

It took me most of my life to realize (and it still takes consistent reminders to remember) the truth I've mentioned several times here already: our bodies and souls should be one, not two parts, but one united person. Saint Paul points this out in 1 Corinthians 6:19–20 (although I only really understood it this way recently): "Do you not know that your body is a temple of the Holy Spirit within you, which you have from God? You are not your own; you were bought with a price. So glorify God in your body." He's speaking of a union of body and spirit; that's what makes the temple. We belong to God; we are not our own. Through his death on the cross, Jesus bought us at a great price. The good news is, he bought us away from death, from the separation of body and soul that God never intended.

We'll suffer both in body and soul, in small ways and big ways, not only when we do things that are bad for us, but also when we do the things that are good for us. Remember, that's something Adam and Eve earned for us through original sin — that even the things that are good for us bring suffering. With their disobedience, work (which is good for us) became burdensome, food (which is good for us) took toil to acquire, man's and woman's desire for each other (which is good for us) became easily distorted, and even giving new life came only through great pains in childbirth. And because our wills are weakened and our intellects dimmed, doing what's good in every capacity became more difficult.

Living for God and dying to self is challenging. But in Christ we have an opportunity to offer every single suffering back to him so that he can transform it to help us grow, to change us, to bring us closer to him. So don't run away from suffering, especially the suffering that comes from doing the things that are good for you. Embrace it. Conquer your fear, laziness, anger, gluttony, lust, all the things that keep you incomplete, and master your body, mind, and soul. Then the suffering you're bound to experience anyway will serve our mission: a life lived out by our souls through our bodies — one in which we can know, love, and serve God.

CHAPTER THREE
Virtue and the Power of Habit

"He who combines the practice of the virtues with spiritual knowledge is a man of power. For with the first he withers his desire and tames his incensiveness [his tendency to excite or provoke], and with the second he gives wings to his intellect and goes out of himself to God."

— Saint Maximus the Confessor

There's a truism that people only change out of "inspiration or desperation," and I remember a therapist I know once saying: "For someone to change for the better, they don't have to love the good. They don't even have to want to love the good. All they have to do is want to want to love the good. God can work with that." As he pointed out, the bar to start positive change is actually very low. So, if you find yourself in a place of mind, body, heart, or soul that you're unhappy about… good. Otherwise you have no inspiration (or point of desperation) from which to effect change. G. K. Chesterton puts the question this way: "Can [you] hate it enough to change it, and yet love it enough to think it worth changing?"

In the fall of Adam and Eve, our nature was corrupted. As a result, all of humanity experiences a weakened will, so that we all totally relate when Saint Paul says: "I do not understand my own actions. For I do not do what I want, but I do the very thing I hate" (Rom 7:15). We struggle to figure out our lives, and even after we do we struggle to live them. The good news is that in Jesus Christ we receive the grace to reorient our actions and our desires toward the right things, toward things that are truly good — and don't just look good. It's a fascinating little principle of life that, very frequently, we first have to consistently orient our actions to the good before our desires are oriented toward the good.

So, what does all this have to do with virtue? Well, virtues are the qualities of spirit that enable us to choose the good. More specifically, the *Catechism of the Catholic Church* says: "A virtue is an habitual and firm disposition to do the good. It allows the person not only to perform good acts, but to give the best of himself … he pursues the good and chooses it in concrete actions" (1803).

Virtues, both natural and supernatural, come to us most readily as the product of habit. Remember the anecdote of a woman praying to be more patient and loving? Rather than knocking her free will out of the way and transforming her into a caricature of kindness, God provided her plentiful opportunities to *practice* patience and kindness. Far more challenging (but also better). Practicing virtue (natural and supernatural), and *consistently* practicing it, and habitually choosing the good, are the only sure ways to stop neglecting what is truly good for our souls and/or our bodies.

What does that look like? Well, to my mind, that means a daily practice of *exercising* your heart and soul, body and mind, coupled with a daily practice of *feeding* your heart and soul, body and mind. A daily practice of giving your heart and soul, body and mind the rest they need. In the workout guides at the end of this book, I've provided what you'll need to create a daily practice, one that stays dynamic from one day to the next, and uses each day as preparation for the next. But as I mentioned earlier, the only way even a plan for single day works is if you do it. Then do it again the second day. Then do it again the third day. Take it one day at a time, but let that day always be from today until tomorrow.

Your daily practice stretches from this very minute for the next twenty-four hours, not the past twenty-four. What are you doing right now and in the next twenty-four hours to live in accord with the truth, with your goals, with your greatest good? What action will you take in this moment to do the difficult but necessary thing? That's the question always before us: Will I choose the slide of easy counterfeits, or the harder climb of authentic virtue? There are a million temptations, excuses, and unhealthy desires that can derail us. The key is to exercise both your mind and your free will to say, "I see that for what it is, and I choose the good instead."

When I'm busy or sick, or have sinned, I know I'm tempted to say, "If I don't really pray today, that's fine, I prayed yesterday," or "I'll pray tomorrow, that's good enough." The truth is God doesn't need my prayers, I do. When I'm busy or sick or frustrated, I know I'm tempted to say: "This sin will make me feel better… and it's so little. It doesn't really matter. I'm good enough." The truth is God doesn't need me to be good, I do. When I'm busy or sick or tired, I know I'm tempted to say: "I can skip my workout. I'm too tired to do it well anyway. It doesn't matter this one time," or "I know it's not good for me to eat another half loaf of bread in fondue, but it's not a big deal. It's fine." The truth is God doesn't need me to treat the temple of my body with respect… I do.

What we do today with our bodies and our souls is what we do tomorrow with our bodies and souls, unless we make a change and keep reorienting ourselves toward that change. I have a good friend who was in really peak physical condition. He ate right, exercised regularly and well, and made sure to get enough sleep. Then a particularly frustrating and stressful holiday season arrived. First his eating well fell by the wayside. It's an easy temptation between Thanksgiving and Christmas. He continued to struggle all the way until Easter. By Pentecost, fifty days later, he'd created a six-month habit of poor eating. All the while, there was so much to do, so much traveling, so much work to fit in, and then the time he had set aside for workouts and for proper sleep started to vanish. Now, it's been three years, and I'll still hear him say: "I'm going to get back to eating right and working out. Let's start Monday!" Then, if you haven't guessed, Monday comes, but Sunday was a late night, and the gym is deprived of his presence again. Remember, this was one of my most in-shape, peak-physical-condition friends!

The fact is, we can't practice virtue of any kind "on Monday." There is no Monday, there is no "next week," there is no "my New Year's resolution will be …" when it comes to virtue. We only have one actual moment in which to choose the good, and that is right now. If we choose poorly now, it becomes easier to choose poorly again. But if we choose well right now, it becomes easier to choose well in the next moment, and the next moment after that, and the next moment after that. To paraphrase the *Catechism*, we build habit and firm disposition to do what's good. This habitual doing good allows us not only to perform good acts, but to give the best of ourselves. Eventually, we pursue the good because we begin to love it and more easily choose it in concrete actions. That's virtue, lived out in our souls and through our bodies. So… do it!

CHAPTER FOUR
Where Two or Three are Gathered

"Order your soul; reduce your wants; live in charity; associate in Christian community; obey the laws; trust in Providence."

— Saint Augustine

Our need for other people is a central mystery that we can deeply relate to on a natural level. Four centuries before Christ, Aristotle recognized our need for others when he wrote, "Man is a political animal." Loneliness — that lack of real and deep relationships — can break our hearts and sap our strength. Conversely, when we have a friend, a confidante, to rely on and share with, our joys can be magnified, our sorrows lessened, our failings nipped in the bud, and our successes repeated.

Throughout Scripture, too, we read of the power and importance of friends, of community, of fellow believers:

- "It is not good that the man should be alone; I will make him a helper fit for him" (Gn 2:18).
- "And though a man might prevail against one who is alone, two will withstand him. A threefold cord is not quickly broken" (Eccl 4:12).
- "A friend loves at all times, / and a brother is born for adversity" (Prv 17:17).
- "Iron sharpens iron, / and one man sharpens another" (Prv 27:17).
- "For where two or three are gathered in my name, there am I in the midst of them" (Mt 18:20).

As humans, we are created in the image of God, and as Saint John reveals in 1 John 4:8: "God is love." God is, in his very nature, love; the Trinity is an eternal communion of persons. This, according to the *Catechism*, is "the central mystery of Christian faith and life" (234).

In our spiritual lives, we may (or may not!) recognize the importance of church, of praying with others, of seeking spiritual directors, or of having accountability partners to help us live a life of virtue and avoid sin. Each of these bring us deeper into the two great commandments: love of God and love of neighbor. What better way to love God than in and through our neighbor? And truly, if you are set on avoiding sin and growing in virtue, having a like-minded friend with whom you can share mutual accountability can transform the strength of your resolve.

When it comes to exercise and fitness, we similarly set ourselves up for success when we share a human connection in the practice of it. Camaraderie and friendly competition can transform fitness from something on a must-do list into something we look forward to each day.

I have a handful of friends I really look forward to working out with, and they pull me out of slumps when I'm (as I mentioned in the previous chapter) busy or sick or tired, and they do that in different ways. When I'm slacking on the discipline of duration, my friend Jeff is always up for a distance run or a long workout. When I'm not eating right, my brothers Josiah and Eli remind me to keep track of my nutrition and change up my habits. When I want to try something different, my friend Joe always has a new plan he's just read about that we can do together. When I know I really need to ramp up my workouts and have my butt kicked, my buddy Hunter is ready (and willing) to do the kicking.

And when either my wife or I feel too busy, we have an "I'll go if you'll go" protocol, so we don't miss out on time together but still take care of ourselves (and each other). The truth is, there are a ton of different ways that training partners can help each other, in both physical and spiritual fitness. There are also some practical needs and benefits.

Accountability: Sometimes you really just need someone to be accountable to, someone who will be there and that you will be letting down if you don't show up (or if you don't give it your all when you do show up).

This is true when it comes to practicing any kind of virtue, be it purity or push-ups (apologies for the cheesy alliteration). Most mothers won't *not* feed their children because they know their children are counting on them. If your training partner is counting on you, chances are much better that you'll show up and work hard.

Two caveats: First, if you're the kind of person who has even a slight habit of no-showing, regularly being more than five minutes late, or trying to cancel things (not just workouts, anything) last minute, then you need to start taking more personal responsibility and put more emphasis on the importance of keeping your word. An accountability partner won't be able to help you, simply because you don't really feel accountable to anyone, even to yourself.

Second, don't pick an accountability partner who will even think about having this conversation with you: "Man, I'm tired out, totally not motivated to do our workout." "I hear you! You know what? Maybe we just skip it today." That's not accountability, that's a millstone around your neck. So be a person of accountability, and find a person who will be the same.

Encouragement: Think back to a difficult moment in your life, one where you felt alone, or like you couldn't do it, or just couldn't make it through. Imagine how different it would have felt to have someone right there with you, someone who had been through the same thing, saying: "You can do this. I know you can do this. You've got it, you're almost done. You're doing so awesome, you got this!"

It may sound silly to compare a difficult workout with a difficult time in your life, but there's more than a superficial correlation. If you work out regularly, and you work out well, I promise you will encounter challenges that you look at and say, "There's no way I can do that." And then, with encouragement, you'll do it.

This principle absolutely translates over to the rest of your life. When you can look at small things you find impossible, small tasks that still seems insurmountable, and then surmount them, you're encouraged and lifted up to tackle the harder things, the bigger moments of life with more faith and more grace.

Spotting: If you are lifting heavy weights, or trying an exercise for the first time, a friend can be a "spotter." A spotter is someone there to watch your form and help you complete the lift if you fail, and it's always better if that person is someone you know and can have consistency with. This allows them to know and see your needs (and vice versa), help just as much as you need and no more, and correct your form on an ongoing basis, based on the knowledge of your strengths, weaknesses, and goals.

I've learned the hard way that not all spotters are created equal. The most major sports injury I've had occurred when I asked a random guy in the gym to spot me, he clearly didn't want to (but knew that gym etiquette dictated that he ought to), and even though I told him the kind of lifting I was doing, which necessitated focused, literally hands-on (on the barbell, not on me, in case there was any confusion) attention, he didn't follow through on any part of it, and I ended up tearing a muscle. Know your spotter, or pick a different kind of workout until you find a spotter. And, when you are needed to spot someone else, be attentive.

Competition: If you're someone who even remotely enjoys games or, you know, fun, at all, getting fitter with a training partner becomes much easier. I have some friends with whom I switch off coming up with workouts, and we see who can do it better, or faster, or longer. It's fun to push through your plateaus, to challenge your strengths and your weaknesses, and to share all of that with a friend.

The adage of "if you're the smartest person in the room, you're in the wrong room" holds true here. I have friends who are stronger than I am, friends who are faster than I am, friends who have better endurance, friends who are more flexible, friends who excel at a certain sport. All of them can drive me to show up and do my best, with the hopes that one day my best might beat them!

Learning: I mentioned earlier that my friend Joe always has a new workout he's just read about and is excited to try. The truth is, most of my training partners are constantly learning and trying new things, whether it be with nutrition, exercise, rest, discipline, skill training, etc. Two heads really are better than one.

When I train with them, I'm constantly learning new things, and that helps me come up with new goals, new ways of reaching my current goals, or new skills I want to develop. Most people resist change, but we also thrive on change. If the person who's keeping you accountable can also provide a source of learning and potential growth for you, positive change becomes easier. That's gold.

Wow, look how great training partners can be! Who knew? "Who" is indeed the right question, because that leads us to the final topic in this section: how to find training partners. There are a multitude of different ways to approach this, but here I'll present a few, along with some other things to keep in mind.

Start talking more about the things that are important to you. (For purposes of our discussion, those would be faith and fitness). Back in 2013, pretty much immediately after finishing my first Spartan Race, when people asked "what's up?" or "what's new?" I'd tell them, "I'm really getting into obstacle racing." I had done one race! And I hadn't even done very well. But I was excited about it, and that was exciting to others. It made some other friends comfortable enough to say things like: "You know, I've thought about doing that, but didn't know who I'd train with. Want to go for a trail run some time?" We found a new common bond and started training together. The same holds true for when I first started getting into my faith. It became a go-to topic for me and made others comfortable enough to dialogue about it and dive deeper.

Ask just outside your most immediate circle of friends. Chances are if you have a friend in your immediate circle of friends who is at a similar point of wanting to get fitter and better across the board, they're already your training partner. If they're not, well, for heaven's sake, ask them. More likely though, if you've been talking about fitness and haven't found an immediate friend who's interested, you need to cast a wider net.

I can think of several times in my life when I had a particular fitness goal (in one instance it was endurance running), and I was making mention of it to pretty much all of my immediate friends. One finally said: "You know, you should talk to my friend Yanni. He used to run all the time. I think he still does. He'd probably be down to train together." So I talked to him, he said he was always looking for a new running buddy, and we started running together.

So, ask others for recommendations. Even if you don't feel comfortable bugging all your friends about their friends, try posting on Facebook that you're looking for folks who want to train together. People will come out of the woodwork. I do recommend (whether it's on faith or fitness), trying to focus Facebook posts so that it's an invitation to specific training or accountability, etc. This prevents the all-too-common: "Man, there's ANOTHER post from Kaiser. Does he do ANYTHING other than post about obstacle racing and Catholicism? Tuning him out!" It's that syndrome that can happen when people feel bombarded by someone's Facebook feed. And, as in all things social, don't throw safety to the wind. Be smart about who, where, and when you plan to meet someone you don't know really well.

Train for something in particular. Here's another example from my own experience. Before obstacle racing, I had only one occasional training partner. When I started training for my second race, like I recommended above, I posted about it on Facebook. Suddenly, I had someone to train with every day of the week. Friends who wanted to run, acquaintances who wanted to lift, people who wanted to train specifically for obstacle racing and didn't know how into it I was. (By the time I registered for my second race, I had stopped talking about how I was "getting into" obstacle racing, and had moved on to "I obstacle race.")

Now, I have friends of friends who say, "Hey, I heard you were into obstacle racing, wanna train together?" The same proves true for friends who mention frequently or publicly that they're training for a marathon (heck, even a 5k!), starting a CrossFit class, cycling, or rock climbing. If you pick a sport, or an event, and talk publicly about it or post about it on social media, I promise you'll find other people who are doing the same, even among people you're kind of already friends with and can get along with.

Even if you don't find them immediately, do the event or the sport or the class. Some of my training partners are people I've met at a race, sometimes even during the race. I pass them or they pass me, and at the finish we end up introducing ourselves!

Find someone better than you. In general, you want someone who's going to push you. Ideally, you can find someone who's either, like, 10% better than you, or is better in one area but you're better in another. Basically, if someone's a 100% better athlete than you, they're not necessarily going to get much out of being training partners, so it probably won't work long term. But if they're a little better than you, you can probably still give each other the push, the encouragement, and the competition that will help you both thrive. Or, if you have complementary skill sets, you can both challenge each other's weaknesses with your strengths and create a really dynamic environment.

My friend Jeff is a much better runner than I am, but I'm stronger than he is. When we train together, we push each other outside of our wheelhouses to grow and be better. Again, the same holds true in our faith lives. Find people who embody a virtue or a spiritual life that inspires you. Spend more time with them, talk with them, and grow with them and from them.

So, in faith and in fitness, finding a "training partner" keeps us encouraged, accountable, and striving to get better, do better, and be better. But to get to "better" means that not only must we have a fixed ideal we're progressing toward, we must know specifically where we're starting from. How do we figure that out? Well, read on.

CHAPTER FIVE
The Examen

"The Christian soul knows it needs Divine Help and therefore turns to him
Who loved us even while we were yet sinners. Examination of conscience, instead
of inducing morbidity, thereby becomes an occasion of joy."
— Servant of God Archbishop Fulton J. Sheen

Pretty much every fitness company, resource, or book (this one included) will encourage you to both talk to a physician or other medical professional before beginning a fitness program, as well as take a close and serious look at your life to see where you're starting from, and where you want to get to. Unfortunately, when people start a fitness program, they nearly always start based on where they wish they were physically, rather than where they really are.

Saint Ignatius of Loyola begins his Spiritual Exercises by recommending we start every day with an Examen, an examination of our conscience. It forces us to pause a moment, be honest with ourselves as to what our current state of our life is, draw awareness to what sins and imperfections we are fighting, and consciously resolve to improve those that day. He then says that we should do a second examination around midday and a third at night, so that throughout the day we are checking in with ourselves and God to see where we are, and where we need to be.

Saint Ignatius's call to us to examine our consciences and spiritual lives daily echoes throughout our Catholic tradition. As early as the writing of 1 Corinthians (11:27–31, if you want to get specific) Saint Paul calls for, at minimum, a weekly examination of our lives to discern whether we are in a state of grace sufficient to receive holy Communion. Likewise, a competent spiritual director will help us take an honest inventory of where we are before suggesting where we need to grow and how we might do that.

As far as prayer and the spiritual life go, in this book I've tried to incorporate things into the text and the "workouts" that all can benefit from, and yet most of us don't do. But, in almost no realm of life is there such a thing as a "one-size-fits-all" solution. So, it's always good to seek the guidance of a competent pastor, spiritual director, deacon, religious brother or sister, or lay minister.

But when it comes to fitness, how can we figure out where we are starting from? When I used to work as a personal trainer, I would always have clients start by telling me about any injuries, surgeries, etc., they had had. In the case of joint replacements, major hospitalizations, or entire muscles being removed or permanently altered, get the help of a professional physical therapist. There are ways to heal our bodies from almost any starting point, but you will need something a little more custom-tailored.

Here I'm going to break down starting points in general fitness, strength, speed, endurance, and flexibility so you can have a working idea of where to begin.

I. GENERAL FITNESS

How do I feel? This may seem like a silly or woo-woo question, but it's actually a pretty good starting place. If you're honest with yourself, do you feel like you're a beginner, intermediate, or advanced athlete? Does the word athlete intimidate you, feel good when you try it on for size, or do you scoff at it? (In which case, come on, let's calm down on the pride front a little bit here.) Again, be honest.

How long has it been since I worked out regularly? If the answer is "never" to "one year ago," consider yourself a beginner. Every opportunity you have to take pride out of the equation, do it. You can always progress more quickly if beginner stuff feels too easy.

Heart rate. One other important measure to be aware of is your "maximum heart rate." This can be a great metric in any of your fitness training. There are more precise ways to calculate it, but the simplest is 220 beats per minute (bpm) minus your age. So, if you're thirty years old, your "maximum heart rate" is 190 bpm.

Your maximum heart rate becomes important because during different kinds of training, you may have a goal of pushing to 80–90% maximum heart rate, 50–60% heart rate, etc., depending on what skills you're trying to develop.

When you're training, if you do have a heart-rate goal, you'll need to check it. To do so, pause what you're doing and place two fingers on your carotid artery on the right side of your neck. Count how many beats/pulses you feel in 20 seconds, then multiply by 3. You can do a 10-second count and multiply by 6, but 20 seconds is a little easier to be accurate. Obviously the most accurate way is to get a heart-rate monitor that you wear, but you can do that if and when you feel ready for it.

II. STRENGTH

A. The Pull-up/Push-up/Squat test. These three movements serve as a great way to gauge where your strength level is, because together they work pretty much every muscle in your body.

1. FEMALE BEGINNERS:
   a) 0–1 pull-ups
   b) 0–5 push-ups
   c) Squat < 50% bodyweight for 8 reps

2. MALE BEGINNERS:
   a) 0–2 pull-ups
   b) 0–10 push-ups
   c) Squat < 50% bodyweight for 8 reps

3. FEMALE INTERMEDIATE
   a) 1–5 pull-ups
   b) 5–15 push-ups
   c) Squat 50–75% bodyweight for 8 reps

4. MALE INTERMEDIATE
   a) 2–10 pull-ups
   b) 10–30 push-ups
   c) Squat 50–100% bodyweight for 8 reps

5. FEMALE ADVANCED
   a) > 5 pull-ups
   b) > 15 push-ups
   c) Squat > 75% bodyweight for 8 reps

6. MALE ADVANCED
   a) > 10 pull-ups
   b) > 30 push-ups
   c) Squat > 100% bodyweight for 8 reps

B. As in the general fitness section, you should also factor in frequency of workouts into your calculations.

III. SPEED

A. 1-mile time. If we're talking overall fitness, your 1-mile time is a pretty good measure of the speed component. It doesn't really take into account your starting/stopping/plyometric speed, but it gives us an idea of how well your body is processing lactic acid buildup (an acid that your body produces when you exert yourself, that makes it more challenging to continue to exert yourself) and your current level of cardiovascular fitness.

1. FEMALE BEGINNER
a)   Can't complete a mile — 12-minute mile

2. MALE BEGINNER
a)   Can't complete a mile — 10-minute mile

3. FEMALE INTERMEDIATE
a)   12-minute mile — 8-minute mile

4. MALE INTERMEDIATE
a)   10-minute mile — 6-minute mile

5. FEMALE ADVANCED
a)   Sub 8-minute mile

6. MALE ADVANCED
a)   Sub 6-minute mile

IV. ENDURANCE

A. Time. The most consistent metric to use to measure your endurance level is how long you can maintain an elevated heart rate without needing to rest. I tend to use 75–80% of maximum heart rate (oh, look, it's already becoming important!). Here the time is the same for both males and females. You'll see there is a large range, and that's because we're talking endurance, the ability to exert yourself for a long time. You could even divide up the advanced section into multiple brackets, but these serve as good starting places.

1. BEGINNER
  a) < 1 minute — 20 minutes

2. INTERMEDIATE
  a) 20 minutes — 90 minutes

3. ADVANCED
  a) > 90 minutes

V. FLEXIBILITY

A. In the included workouts, flexibility will be the only component that doesn't categorize you as beginner, intermediate, or advanced. Wherever you start, you will end up doing the same amount of flexibility work. But it is important to get a clear idea of where you're starting from, so here are good ways to check. Bonus: most of them double as pretty good stretches for flexibility training when we get to workouts!

1. SINGLE LEG FLOOR TOUCH TEST (100); TWO-LEGGED VARIETY (101) With this test, you are checking for imbalance between your hamstrings and back — and the ability to hold a position, rather than getting there by bouncing or quick movement. In the case of flexibility, bouncing is both dangerous and can lead to muscle pulls, strains, and tears.

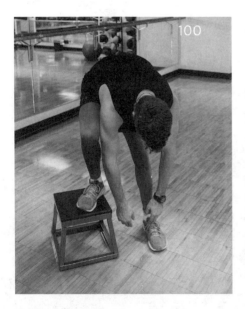 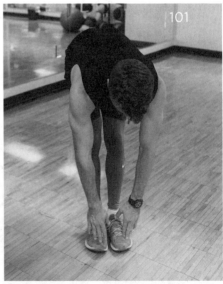

a) Find a short stool (6–10 inches high)
b) Put one foot on the stool, keep the other leg straight, and reach slowly for the foot on the floor with both hands
c) Hold the stretch for 10 seconds at a time
d) Switch sides

2. GROIN FLEXIBILITY TEST (102)

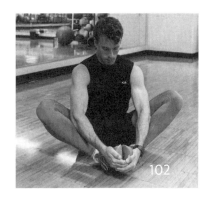

a) Sit on the floor, with knees to each side and feet together
b) Pull your heels back toward your groin, keeping your feet together
c) See how close to your groin you can pull your feet without significant discomfort

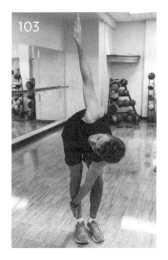

3. TRUNK TWIST (103)

a) Standing in a bent over position, place your left hand on the outside of your right leg
b) Reach your right arm up toward the ceiling while opening up your body to the right side
c) Hold where you begin to experience discomfort for 10 seconds
d) Switch sides

4. BACK SCRATCH TEST (104, 105)

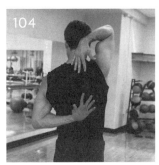

a) Reaching back over your shoulder with one arm, place your fingertips on your back
b) Reaching the other arm behind

your back, place the knuckles
on the back

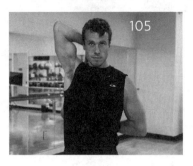

c) Try to bring both hands to touch
d) Preferably, have a partner measure the
distance between your hands so
you can gauge it
e) Switch sides and repeat

Okay, so those are ways to discern where you are starting from. Again, each one, the point is just to get a clear idea of where you are beginning. You may be ahead in one category and behind in another. You may be significantly ahead or behind of where you expected to be in a category, or overall. No matter what the circumstances, resist the temptation to despair or to be too self-satisfied. Both come from pride, and both will inhibit the possibility for real learning, growth, and change.

PART 2
The Components of Fitness

CHAPTER SIX
Strength

"Having faith does not mean having no difficulties, but having the strength to face them, knowing we are not alone."

— Pope Francis

The foundation of any physical fitness program is strength building, plain and simple. "But I don't want to get too big," you say. There are two answers to that.

One: Seriously, do you think you're going to go to bed one night in the body you're used to and wake up the next morning as a human tank? Growth, generally speaking, happens gradually, and there will be no Hulk transformations, I promise.

Two: Size and strength are not synonymous. The goal of this chapter is to help you find an appropriate level of strength to meet your needs and desires. "But I can't lift weights... I have injuries!" you cry. Wow, you're full of excuses today. I promise we'll address them. But first, let's start with why strength training is so important.

Literally every part of physical fitness involves strength in some capacity. From the beginning, Genesis tells us that God makes us in his own image, to share in the act of creation, to have dominion over the earth and subdue it (see Gn 1:26–28). Apparently, that's hard enough work that even God himself takes the seventh day to rest! God doesn't give us any capacity or gift to be left unused. As Jesus reveals in the parable of the talents (Mt 25:14–30), and like we discussed in Chapter Three on virtue, every repetition of good action builds our ability to repeat good action in the future. Similarly, God created our bodies to respond to work and stress by growing stronger as well. Noticing a pattern at all?

It bears repeating that since God made us a unity of body and spirit, there are generally cognates in the physical life that directly mirror the spiritual life. Any good spiritual action will produce growth in strength of virtue, and physical actions will result in more basic physical strength.

Obviously, this applies to the other fitness components as well. Speed necessitates strong fast-twitch muscle fibers; endurance requires strong slow-twitch muscle fibers; flexibility requires pliability and isometric strength. But this also applies to our daily lives. As my friend Carlen says, "What's the point of fitting into a size zero dress if I can't carry my groceries?"

From sitting at a desk all day, to standing behind a counter, to doing housework or work around the house, to wrangling kids and running errands, to enjoying leisure indoors or outdoors, we use our muscles every single minute of every single day, and if they're stronger, our physical lives will be easier, more relaxing, and more enjoyable. Perhaps most importantly (and often most overlooked), strong muscles actually help to prevent injuries that take us away from the lives we want to live.

This all holds true in our spiritual lives, too: When we focus on the big questions of strengthening our relationship with God, the details take care of themselves. As an example, I heard a priest say once that when it comes to purity, if you can focus on the good of God's intent for sex (a full, faithful, fruitful, and forever gift of self for the good of the other), that's what will become appealing, and everything else will fall to the wayside. If we train our souls and our bodies to do the good, the smaller aspects of it fall into place, and the smaller symptoms of our inclinations away from the good fade out.

Saint Augustine said, "Love, and do what you will." If our minds, hearts, bodies, and souls are fervently loving God and neighbor, our desires will be oriented toward only the good and virtuous. If we are strong and devoted in our spiritual lives, temptations still occur, but they don't master us. If we are strong and devoted in our spiritual lives, even when we fall, we long for communion with God so much that we rapidly seek to heal our relationship with him.

So, let's get into the most fundamental component of fitness. We'll look at some of the best ways to strength train, and then we'll wrap up with how to use that training to recover from injury and prevent it in the first place.

Olympic Lifting and Powerlifting

If you've watched the Olympics, you've seen competitive weightlifters throwing terrifying amounts of weight over their heads in various ways. If you've watched strongman competitions, you've seen guys picking up cars, barrels, and other absurdly heavy stuff, and setting it back down until they can't do it anymore. The commonalities here are that many of these lifts are heavy compound movements that involve most of the body and take it through a natural range of motion.

They're not doing crunches, calf raises, forearm curls, or anything of the sort. Yet, these lifters all have absurdly strong abs, calves, and forearms (as well as every other muscle in the body). Again, just as in the spiritual life, when we focus on the big things, the little ones take care of themselves.

In the last couple of years, this style of lifting has become my favorite style of lifting, and it's catching on nationwide and worldwide as evidenced by the CrossFit craze. Why? It works. It's a rapid way to gain strength, and if done properly, builds your body in a way that helps prevent injury because, again, it's taking you through a natural range of motion.

I. WHAT ARE THE MAIN CONCEPTS?

A. HEAVY WEIGHT
1. The whole point is to use a weight that is difficult, something that challenges you. The first few times you do the lifts, start light so that you can develop proper technique. But some lifts will be hard to get right without at least some significant weight.

B. LOW REPS/EXPLOSIVE MOVEMENT
1. It's called "powerlifting" for a reason! You're developing explosive strength. Endurance will come later. I'll almost never perform more than 7 reps in a set. Usually I'll do 3–5. If you think you'll risk compromising your form by doing another rep, don't do the rep.

C. FEW SETS
1. These lifts will work multiple major muscle groups at once. While workout plans you may have encountered before might have you doing 9–15 sets for one muscle group, these lifts don't need that. You will reach the maximum work you really need within 3–8 sets. The larger the muscle group, the more sets. So, for example, if I'm working legs and shoulders, I might do 5 sets of squats and 3 of clean and jerk, and then I'm done lifting for the day. That basically gives me 8 sets for legs (both exercises work legs), 3 sets for shoulders (the clean and jerk works legs, back, arms, and shoulders), which is totally sufficient.

D. BIG REST BETWEEN SETS

1. After doing big, explosive, compound movements, your whole body needs to recover. Rest for 2–3 minutes between each set. Seriously. Just rest.

E. DON'T GO TO FAILURE

1. Don't let yourself off easy and stop when it starts to get hard; the whole set should be challenging. But don't go to the point where you can't complete the rep. Stop 1–2 reps before that would happen. If you have a coach and you're training for a weightlifting competition, he or she can take you to failure safely. Most of the time, however, there's no need to do that with these kinds of lifts, and it's safer to stop before failure.

II. WHAT ARE THE MAIN LIFTS?

A. OLYMPIC LIFTS
1. Clean and jerk
2. Snatch

B. POWER LIFTS
1. Bench
2. Dead lift
3. Squat

C. MORE OF A FEW OF MY FAVORITE LIFTS
1. Front squat
2. Clean and press
3. Thruster

D. Just a reminder, all of these lifts (in fact, all the lifting, stretching, and exercise techniques in the book) will be covered in more detail in the workout section (Part III).

High Intensity Training

High Intensity Training (HIT) shares some crossover with powerlifting, but also departs from it in certain ways. High intensity training is more of a training style than simply the type of lifts you're doing. The main idea is to fully exhaust the muscle to the point of muscle failure through brief, infrequent (meaning each muscle group usually only gets exercised once a week, maximum), but intense work. This can be applied to nearly any specific exercise, but most plans will start with a compound muscle exercise, followed by an isolation exercise for each muscle group. For instance, if you were working your chest and biceps, you might do bench press (which works chest, triceps, and shoulders) followed by flyes (which isolates chest), then barbell curl (which involves back, shoulders, biceps, and forearms), followed by dumbbell hammer curl (which more directly targets your biceps and forearms alone).

I. WHAT ARE THE MAIN CONCEPTS?

A. HEAVY WEIGHT
1. You're trying to fully exhaust your muscles quickly, so you will be moving some good weight! Again, start light to develop proper technique, but after that, be sure to challenge yourself.

B. MEDIUM REPS/CONTROLLED MOVEMENT
1. Execute your compound lifts (bench, dead lift, row, squat, etc.) in a 6–8 rep range and your isolation lifts in an 8–10 rep range. Reps go slow and controlled: 2–4 seconds in the contraction of the rep, 4 seconds in the negative portion of the rep. Count it out. It's easy to go too fast.

C. ONE SET
1. Just one set per exercise, maximum 2–3 exercises per major muscle group. That's it.

D. REST BETWEEN WORKOUTS
1. There are no long rests between sets here, because each exercise only has one set. You can rest for a max of 1 minute between exercises, and that's it. But don't work the same muscle group again for at least 5 days or, even better, rest a full week. So, if you work chest on Monday (but don't, because everyone works chest on Mondays), don't work it again until about next Monday.

E. GO TO FAILURE
1. Your reps are slow and controlled so, where it is safe to, feel free to push until failure. Obviously, that will depend on whether you have a training partner and what lift you're doing (for example, if you're doing bench without a training partner, save failure for your set of flyes). But the goal here is to fully exhaust

the muscle, so, in general, every exercise should end in failure at your desired rep range.

WODs, EMOMs, AMRAPs

I know, they sound like weapons, but WODs (which usually are either an EMOM, an AMRAP, or For Time) serve as a great way to take your functional strength to the next level.

WOD simply stands for "Workout of the Day." This term is taken from CrossFit, where classes involve everyone doing the same workout challenge. While sometimes I'll do a WOD as my only workout (see Knockin' on Heaven's Door in the workout supplement), usually I'll start with some powerlifting and then do a short WOD afterward. This is often how CrossFit classes do it as well. Those workout challenges usually takes one of the following forms:

I. EMOM (EVERY MINUTE ON THE MINUTE)
A. In an EMOM, usually you pick two exercises and perform them on alternating minutes (for example, 5 pull-ups on minutes 0, 2, 4, 6, and 8, and 15 squats on minutes 1, 3, 5, 7, and 9). You can include more exercises or choose a longer amount of time if you like, but 2 exercises and 10 minutes is a great starting point.

II. AMRAP (AS MANY REPS AS POSSIBLE)
A. In an AMRAP, you pick a certain amount of time and complete as many times through a circuit as you can before the time expires. So, you may have a 2 or 3 exercise circuit, and do it as many times as possible in 10 minutes. Or if you're feeling ambitious, or aren't doing any other lifting, you might try one with 5 or 6 exercises and up to 30 minutes long. There are people who do 60 minute AMRAPs, but my philosophy is that almost nobody can push for a whole hour as hard as you're supposed to push in an AMRAP.

III. FOR TIME
A. When you're doing a WOD "For Time" you complete one workout as fast as you can… then tell everyone how fast you did it on every conceivable form of social media. One of the most famous For Time workouts is named "Murph," after U.S. Navy Lieutenant Michael Murphy, killed in Afghanistan in 2005, who prized it as one of his favorite workouts. It involves running 1 mile; completing 100 pull-ups, 200 push-ups, and 300 squats; and running 1 more mile, as quickly as you can. There are certainly easier ones to start with, but Murph is the

quintessential For Time workout.

Strength Training Without Weights

"Well, Powerlifting, HIT, and all those acronyms sound great, but I don't have a gym membership!" Okay, go get one.

"I live in an old monastery, 100 miles from the nearest town, and can't afford to buy weights because I've taken a vow of poverty!" Wow, that's a very specific set of circumstances. Lucky for you, I have several ways you can still get your strength training in.

After all, strong people existed long before ubiquitous access to barbells, dumbbells, and kettlebells… because there are plenty of other heavy things to lift. My friend Josh actually lived in a monastery for a while, and his workouts consisted of a handful of lifts he could do with a log he found. In my Obstacle Course Race (OCR) training, I frequently use a sandbag or two (usually free for the asking at any local fire station) and an old truck tire. Get creative and use objects you can find to get your strength training in! Sometimes the simplest "found object" is just your body.

Here are a couple of my favorite exercises if I've just got my own weight (body) to lift. Descriptions and photos are in Part III, "The Workouts."

I. WHOLE BODY
   A. Burpees
   B. 8-count Bodybuilders

II. CHEST, SHOULDERS AND TRICEPS
   A. Push ups
   B. Handstand push up

III. BACK AND BICEPS
   A. Pull ups
   B. Inverted push up

IV. LEGS
   A. Squats
   B. Pistol squats

V. ABS AND CORE
   A. Plank
   B. One-arm plank
   C. Side plank
   D. Plank push-ups
   E. Crunches
   F. Mountain climbers

Injuries

When people ask me about my fitness regimen, a common response I hear goes something like this: "Oh, I could never do that. I mean, not anymore. I used to be in great shape a few years ago/in college/in high school/when I was first born, but then I hurt my back/knees/shoulder/pride, so now I can't even look at a dumbbell without risk to my health."

What people often don't realize is that that makes about as much sense as saying, "Oh, I used to live a virtuous life, but I sinned pretty badly, so now I can't go to confession, much less get my life back on track." The fact is, just as we often fall down in our spiritual lives and need the grace to pick up and start in again, anyone even remotely serious about fitness will experience injury.

The best way to recover nearly always involves specifically training the muscle that is injured, or training the muscles around a joint that was injured. For example, I've tweaked my back while training over-exhausted shoulders. When you get that twinge next to your spine, most people will leave the gym immediately, some never to return. What I do is jump right in to doing pull-ups, which will put my back through a natural range of motion. Nine times out of ten, this instantly corrects the potential injury.

Similarly, folks who avoid squats for the rest of their lives because they've had knee issues often wonder why they're plagued by even more knee injuries, usually while doing minor tasks. If they focused on strengthening the muscles that surround the knee, by putting them through controlled strength-building exercises, like, say, you know, for instance, properly executed squats, they'd experience much faster healing and reduce the likelihood of further injury.

Take a look at athletes. When they are injured, they work closely with a trainer specifically to train the affected area. So when it comes to injury, the key isn't stopping exercise forever; in fact, that compounds the problem. The key is minimizing the frequency of injury and coming back stronger.

Here are the key concepts to both prevention and rehab:

I. PREVENTION

A. EXERCISE KNOWLEDGE
1. Know how to properly execute any exercise you undertake. All the exercises I suggest in this book are laid out in the workout section, and a quick YouTube search will usually yield a multitude of videos demonstrating correct execution. Make sure you're very familiar with any exercise before trying it for the first time.

2. Start light. The first time you perform an exercise (heck, with some of the trickier ones, like snatch, even the second, third, and fourth times) lift a very manageable weight, just to find a natural way to proceed through the movement that feels comfortable to you. Many exercises will need slight adjustments to optimize them for your body. Give yourself the time to feel that out.

B. NEVER GO TOO HEAVY
1. Unless you're training for very specific max effort lifts under the supervision of an expert, never lift a weight with which you will experience muscle failure in less than 5 reps. I'll sometimes do only 3–5 reps of an exercise if I'm doing a powerlifting set, but I'll never have that be the point at which I'm experiencing total muscle failure. Doing that tears muscles. Trust me, I know, because I once tore my chest doing 2-rep sets of heavy bench press.

C. WARM UP AND COOL DOWN
1. Certain muscles and joints are simply more prone to injury; which ones those are often varies from person to person. In general, shoulders and knees and their surrounding muscles tend to be more vulnerable. Whenever I'm exercising those areas, I'll be sure to warm up with light weight and full natural range of motion before doing any serious lifting. If I don't, I know I'm just asking to get injured. Afterward, be sure to stretch and cool down, so your muscles can relax and heal more quickly.

D. TRAIN WITH A PARTNER
1. As we discussed in the previous chapter, partners can help monitor your form, protect you when you are lifting near or at failure, troubleshoot difficult lifts, and in general give you perspective on what they're seeing. A good partner has saved me from injury countless times.

E. DON'T NEGLECT ANY FITNESS COMPONENTS

1. If you neglect flexibility, you'll injure your muscles. If you neglect strength training, you'll injure tendons, joints, and ligaments. If you neglect cardio, well, you'll injure yourself walking up the stairs. Make sure to balance your training, rest, and life.

F. DO EXERCISES THAT TAKE YOUR FULL BODY THROUGH A NATURAL RANGE OF MOTION

1. All exercises should feel like a natural way that your body is made to move. If they don't, find the adjustments to make them work properly. As far as "full body" goes, I'm not saying that every exercise in your workout should involve your whole body. But having at least one full-body exercise in every workout (sometimes both at the beginning as a warm-up and at the end as a cool down), goes a long way to preventing injury. My favorite for that purpose is Turkish Get-Ups. They take some getting used to, but they reset your muscles and joints and whole body unlike anything else I know.

II. REHABBING

A. GET EXPERT HELP

1. That may sound like a cop-out, but if you have seriously injured yourself talk to a physical therapist. Not just your regular doctor, but a physical therapist. This book doesn't have the space (nor, honestly, do I have the expertise) to properly diagnose and treat every possible injury. However, depending on the injury, even a few appointments with a good physical therapist can save you years of pain, struggle, surgeries, and more!

B. DULL ACHING PAIN = OKAY. SHARP STABBING PAIN = BAD.

1. As you rehab any part of your body, there are some kinds of pain that are normal and a good sign of improvement, and some that are just bad. Again, consult an expert, but in general if you are exercising a muscle, dull pain throughout the muscle is totally normal, and to be expected. Sharp stabbing pain, or pain in your joints themselves or right along ligaments or tendons, however, is a bad sign.

Avoid anything that causes that, and troubleshoot the exercise with a professional if you experience it. As an example, the first few times people do dead lifts properly, they will say, "This hurts my back." I then ask, "Is it a sharp stabbing pain in the spine, or a painful ache on either side of the spine?" It's nearly always pain on either side of the spine, which indicates that the spinal erector muscles are being worked properly, maybe for the first time. If it's in the spine, they're doing something with dangerously bad form and need to correct it.

C. TAKE IT EASIER, DON'T STOP

1. Many people make the mistake of avoiding an injured body part entirely, rather than continuing to work it by following the prevention guidelines, which is a recipe for further injury, whether it's a pull, a strain, or even a tear.

For instance, when I tore my chest (my pectorals major, from the middle, through the shoulder, all the way to my bicep, for the record), the physical therapist I saw gave me the following prescription: 2 weeks of complete rest for the chest and shoulder, followed by several weeks of resistance training and very light weights, gradually building to regain full use and regular weights within 4–6 months. This stands in stark contrast to the "well, guess that's the last weight I ever lift" practice of most folks experiencing injuries. Take it easy, but don't shut it down.

So that's the strength training "why and how" in a nutshell. For exercise specifics and how to put it all together, check out Part III.

One final note here. All the concepts that help us avoid physical injury and repair it when it occurs apply to our spiritual lives as well. Expanding our knowledge, having a training/prayer partner and accountability, having expert help from a spiritual director, easing into any spiritual practice, and properly taking care of every aspect of our spiritual lives, all create a much more healthy and vibrant experience and expression of what we believe.

So, if spiritually, you fall down, feel stagnant, or even hurt in some way, take another look at these principles.

CHAPTER SEVEN
Speed

"And after you have suffered a little while, the God of all grace, who has called you to his eternal glory in Christ, will himself restore, establish, and strengthen you."

— 1 Peter 5:10

Like strength training, the ability to exert yourself at a high level for a short period of time can totally and literally transform your health. And when I say "literally," I'm not just using it for emphasis or meaning it metaphorically... thereby using it incorrectly. No, I actually mean "transform" *literally.*

Training your speed recruits your lungs, your heart, and your muscle fibers in ways that no other kind of training does. This, in turn, exponentially increases your efficiency in losing fat, changing your body composition, and improving your cardiovascular function, extending your life and making it easier and more enjoyable.

And yet, almost no one does it! Fewer still do it correctly. Why? Well, it's very taxing. The truth is, most people don't like to work out. It goes against our desire for easy pleasure and our fear of hard work inherited from our original parents.

This is what the Catholic Church calls "concupiscence." If I may draw a comparison to our spiritual lives, G. K. Chesterton tells us, "The Christian ideal has not been tried and found wanting, it has been found difficult and left untried."

Fitness, for both body and soul, is difficult. Working out is work. The truth is that even when we do work out, most of us want to work out just hard enough and just long enough to convince ourselves that we're doing something, rather than truly giving our best effort for an optimal amount of time. It's the difference between activity and intensity. Basically, we exercise too long to maintain a high intensity, or too hard to maintain a long duration. When we get to the endurance chapter, we'll cover the second part of that equation, but when we're talking about harnessing the truly transformative, we're talking about exertion at a much higher intensity for a shorter period of time. That's the proper way to train speed.

What does that look like spiritually? Well, in my experience, I tend to see the most temptation and struggle in my life right when great grace is around the corner. It may be cliché, but it's sometimes as simple as behaving ourselves Saturday night so we're disposed to receive Sunday Communion the next day. I do Saint Louis de Montfort's 33-day consecration each year, and I'll be darned if I don't feel totally dogged by the devil on day 32.

Whether you're preparing for a sacrament like marriage, holy orders, or confirmation, or you're going through Lent or a particularly trying time, your ability to exert yourself at a high intensity in your faith life will open you up to the transformative grace God desires to give you.

As in the strength chapter, I'll discuss the principles of speed in relation to fitness, but most of them are great analogies to growing in faith as well. We'll see that laid out in more detail in the workouts in Part III, but let's get right into the principles.

Sprinting and HIIT

HIIT looks similar to an acronym we saw in the previous chapter, but while HIT stands simply for High Intensity Training, HIIT adds an extra component to become High Intensity Interval Training. Interval training means you incorporate brief intervals of hard work, followed by intervals of either rest or much easier work.

High Intensity (like in the previous chapter) means it should be really, really hard. How hard is really, really hard? Timothy Ferriss, author of *The 4-Hour Body* describes it as, "Pushing like you have a gun to your head." That probably sounds extreme, but in HIIT, you've got to give your all.

This brings us to the concept of sprinting. Sprinting usually refers to running fast for short distances. We can apply the term more generally to mean giving your maximum effort for a very short period of time... one interval. You can do sprints on a track, running up stairs, heck, you can do sprints on a rowing machine or swimming in a pool. Let me show you a few of my favorite ways.

I. TRADITIONAL SPRINTING

A. FIND A GOOD PLACE TO RUN
1. Ideally, it's great to be on a track. It's flat, forgiving, and there are distance markers.

2. A football field works nicely too. It's also flat and fairly forgiving. Once you get to sprinting more than 100 meters though, you'll run out of space and have to turn around.

3. Quiet back streets are okay, but really only the ones that are so little traveled that you'll be able to run straight down the middle to have a fairly even surface. Usually it's difficult to find any that fit the bill over any great distance, so they tend to work best for hill repeats, which we'll get to shortly.

4. Two places to never sprint? Sidewalks and treadmills. When you're sprinting, you want to be able to run as fast as possible, and then just stop and rest immediately. A treadmill, for safety reasons, doesn't allow you to do either of those. Also, most treadmills don't have much give to them, and are very hard on your joints and bones. If your joints and bones aren't used to running, pounding away on a treadmill can be a quick road to injury. Sidewalks are frequently uneven and often made of concrete, which is just about the most unforgiving surface you can run on. I run frequently, and still get sore if I run for any real distance on a sidewalk.

B. LEARN HOW TO RUN

1. There are a lot of schools of thought on the optimal way to run. For our purposes, we're just looking to go fast and avoid injury and are less concerned right now about shaving two-tenths of a second off a 100-meter time. I detail my favorite techniques in Part III, but be sure to find something that works best for you.

C. CHOOSE PROPER FOOTWEAR

1. I can't emphasize this enough. Wear shoes specifically designed for running… not cross-trainers, tennis shoes, basketball shoes, etc. When I first decided I'd start running, I had a clunky old pair of cross-trainers I wore to the gym that I thought "would be fine." They weren't. In a matter of two weeks, I had shin splints and a stress fracture in my left tibia (in the interest of full disclosure, I also was doing most of my running on a treadmill). Go to an athletic shoe store where they check your gait and have them assist you in finding a running shoe that feels good.

2. You can get really specific with track shoes, trail shoes, road shoes, etc., but usually a decent road shoe will suffice for both track and road. We'll cover trail shoes, which actually can make a big difference, in the endurance section.

D. WARM UP

1. Jog for a minimum of 5–10 minutes, work your hip and ankle mobility, and take a couple of minutes to stretch before sprinting. Usually, I'll do a slow mile before I start, as well as a slow "grapevine" walk back and forth.

E. SHORT EFFORT, LONG RECOVERY

1. Remember, we're looking for maximum effort here. Most people (even elite athletes) can only give about 15 seconds of true maximum effort. Start with a little shorter than that, like 10 seconds of maximum effort. You can work up to longer intervals (like 30 seconds or a minute), but those won't really be sprints, because there's no way you can sustain a true maximum effort for that long. So start short, 10–15 seconds, push as hard as you can, then rest and repeat.

2. As far as resting goes, for each interval of effort, rest 2–4 times as long as you exerted yourself. And when you're doing sprinting, it can be total rest. Don't sprint and then jog, just sprint and then stop. For example, if I'm sprinting for 15 seconds, I'll rest for 45 seconds. In the times when I'm working longer intervals, I may run hard for 30 seconds, then rest for 2–2.5 minutes. Ideally, in your rest period, you want your heart rate to drop down to about 60–70% of your maximum heart rate before starting your next sprint. For example, my "max heart rate" is about 190 bpm, so I'll wait until my heart rate drops below 130 bpm, then go again.

F. DON'T DO TOO MANY SPRINTS IN ONE SESSION

1. One way to gauge this is just by limiting your number of intervals. If you're new to sprinting, I would only do 3 intervals. So, that's maximum effort for 10–15 seconds, followed by a 45-second rest. When you get more experienced, bump it up to the 5–7 interval range. But even some of the craziest endurance athletes I've ever trained with still generally limit themselves to 8-10 intervals before calling it quits. This may feel short, but if you do it right, it sure won't feel easy.

2. The second way to gauge a good stopping point is by tracking your distance and time. Let's say it takes you about 15 seconds to run 75 yards on a football field at maximum effort, and so you decide you'll do 7 sprints of 75 yards apiece. But on your fifth sprint, you find that you took almost 20 seconds to make it to 75 yards. You're too fatigued, and it's time to end the workout. Your intervals should stay fairly consistent both in time and in distance. When you sacrifice one or the other, wrap it up.

3. The last way to gauge it will really only come up after you've been training for a while, and that's distance. As a beginner to intermediate, once the total of your intervals adds up to 1 mile (or 1600 meters), even if your intervals are still fine in terms of time and speed, you're good to finish up. If you're really advanced, you may be able to stretch it to double that (2 miles or 3200 meters), but normally even that will be split up into two separate sessions, one at the beginning of a workout, and one at the end.

II. HILL REPEATS

A. FIND A HILL
1. Told you we'd get to this soon! Some people get lucky and live near a big, long hill that goes up at a consistent incline. That's ideal, but all you really need is a stretch of hill that takes you about 15 seconds maximum to run, because again, that's about the most you should be able to do a max effort. You'll then have 3 times as long to jog/walk back down the hill to your starting place.

B. Follow all the rules of traditional sprinting.
    1. Make sure you're running properly
    2. Choose footwear designed for running
    3. Warm up
    4. Rest for 2–3 times as long as you exert max effort
    5. Don't do too many sprints

III. "SPRINTING"

A. PICK AN EXERCISE.
What separates traditional sprinting and "sprinting"? Mainly that, as I mentioned, you can pick almost any cardio exercise to do instead of running. Here are my suggestions:
    1. Bicycle or stationary bike
    2. Stair climber
    3. Rowing machine
    4. Elliptical
    5. Swimming
    6. Running in water

B. Follow the rules. I probably don't have to itemize these again, but here you are:

   1. Make sure you're doing the movement properly

   2. Warm up

   3. Rest for 2–3 times as long as you exert max effort

   4. Don't do too many

IV. DEADMILLS

A. Deadmills are a recently-discovered favorite exercise of mine. In some ways they're easier on your joints, simpler to learn than regular running, and safer to start with if you happen to be carrying extra bodyweight. In addition, they're super-tough, and they take less than 10 minutes. What are they? They're a treadmill exercise that mimics a sled push… the kind you might see football players doing. How do you do them? Simple: you just don't turn on the treadmill. (Which makes it a "deadmill.") Here are the steps.

   1. Get on the treadmill.

   2. After you've warmed up for 2–5 minutes of easy effort, turn the treadmill off (stop the belt from moving).

   3. Lean forward and brace your upper body against the treadmill.

   4. Start a stopwatch or timer.

   5. Push the belt using your feet, for 10–15 seconds as hard as you can.

   6. Stop. Rest for 3 times as long as you pushed. Breathe.

   7. Do it again. Repeat for a total of 3–12 times.

   8. Die. Okay, don't die. But, usually by the time I reach 10 periods of max effort coupled with 10 periods of rest, I am spent, and if I'm lifting that day, it takes me 5–10 minutes to calm my heart rate and breathing down enough to feel like I want to lift. Like I said, they're really tough. If you breeze through 10 of them, you're not pushing yourself (or the belt for that matter) hard enough.

   9. Stretch. You'll likely find your glutes, your calves, and sometimes your quads and hamstrings feeling totally torched. Stretch them out and cool down properly. For more on that, check out the chapter on flexibility.

B. One final thing to be aware of with deadmills: some people have the mistaken impression that they can damage the treadmill by wearing out the motor. If you think about the mechanics of a treadmill or a motor in general, this worry doesn't actually make sense. I have never heard of that actually happening, and there are personal trainers employed by various gyms near me who regularly use deadmills to train their clients without concern. But if you're doing deadmills at your local gym, it's possible someone who's never seen them before might ask you to stop. It's up to you whether you'd like to give them a lesson on basic gear and motor mechanics or not! Or just go into the parking lot and start pushing around cars in neutral. Same basic concept.

So, those are some of my favorite ways to train speed. Again, training speed serves an integral function in changing the way that your body functions to make it more efficient. As your body learns it needs to be able to work your lungs, heart, and muscles at maximum intensity, it quickly finds more and more efficient ways to do that. So get on a track, go up a hill, jump in a pool, hit a bike, or hop on a "deadmill," and go get it!

CHAPTER EIGHT
Endurance

*"Then they will deliver you up to tribulation, and put you to death; and you
will be hated by all nations for my name's sake. And then many will fall away,
and betray one another, and hate one another. And many false prophets will
arise and lead many astray. And because wickedness is multiplied, most men's
love will grow cold. But he who endures to the end will be saved."*

— Matthew 24:9–13

In this passage from Matthew, Jesus offers us a less-than-sunny outlook on
what faithfulness to the Gospel will be rewarded with while we're on earth,
this "vale of tears." It's not enough to be a Christian for a day; what counts is
who's still a Christian on the last day — whether it's our own personal last day,
or the end of the world.

While increasing strength and speed teach us to overcome short-term, high-
level suffering (in addition to the health and well-being benefits they provide),
training our muscular and cardiovascular endurance trains the virtue of long-
suffering. Or maybe better said, the Catholic principle of long-suffering gives us
a glimpse into the importance of physical endurance.

Many of us will go through bouts of intense pain in our lives, but all of us will
experience the long, hard, grind of life much more. If we can learn to appreciate
how that trains our body, mind, and spirit, then when we experience trials
and suffering, we can, as Saint James says: "Count it all joy, my brethren, when
you meet various trials, for you know that the testing of your faith produces
steadfastness. And let steadfastness have its full effect, that you may be perfect
and complete, lacking in nothing" (Jas 1:2–4).

I used to hate running, but after discovering longer obstacle races, I now often
find myself craving a training day when I can just dial into a long slow(er) run…
I relax into the grind, rack up some miles, and just practice the patience (and
sometimes penance!) of putting one foot in front of the other until I finally reach
my destination. How does this benefit us healthwise? Endurance exercise trains

us to push past our perceived physical limitations to recruit muscle fibers, heart and lung capacity, and simple mental grit that we have not yet used. Let's do it.

Distance, Time, and Heart Rate

A lot of people ask what really constitutes endurance training. They wonder whether it's measured in distance or in time, and how hard you have to work. Here are the main concepts:

I. DISTANCE

A. Endurance training can be performed with most types of exercise. You can train endurance through biking, running, walking, hiking, swimming, rowing, and about a hundred other ways — some of which don't have any "distance" associated with them at all! A three-mile hike might take the same time and expend the same amount of calories as a 12-mile run. Consequently, the only occasion where distance is particularly relevant is when you're specifically trying to acclimate your mind and body to doing a certain number of repetitions of an action, like the 55,000 steps it takes on average to complete a marathon.

But a lot of times even that can be accomplished in other ways, and you'll find that many endurance athletes will race a distance for the first time having never run that distance at a race pace in their lives. So, what is the better measure for endurance training? Time.

II. TIME, OR DURATION

A. Along with intensity, which we'll talk about next, duration provides a great metric to help measure the work we're doing in a consistent fashion. I don't consider exercise "endurance training" unless it lasts at least 45 minutes. Longer endurance sessions may last upward of 1–2 hours, or if you're training for an extremely long race, like an ultramarathon or an Ironman-length triathlon, you'll likely need a couple of acclimation training sessions, which usually last about 60–75% of your projected race time.

III. INTENSITY

A. The final component needed to define what we mean by endurance training is intensity. When most people think about endurance training, they're thinking of typical cardiovascular exercise: running, biking, swimming, etc. But to do any of these for an extended period of time takes considerable muscular strength as well. So how do you train your muscles, lungs, heart, and mind to exercise for hours on end? Two main ways: decrease rest and decrease intensity.

1. If you recall from our chapter on strength training, for powerlifting and Olympic lifting, we had short periods of work followed by long periods of rest, and the same principle in our chapter on training speed. In both strength and speed training, we rested for almost 2–3 times the length of time that we exerted effort. When it comes to training endurance, you can almost directly invert that ratio. We'll exert effort for 2–3 times the length of time we rest.

So, for instance, one of my favorite leg endurance workouts involves doing a long set of squats (usually about 2 minutes long) then resting for about 30 seconds before beginning a 90-second wall sit. Obviously, this does force you into using a lighter weight, but it's usually still heavier than you'd imagine you'd be able to do. As a starting point, go for about 60–70% of the weight you would use while doing full-on strength training, and double the length of time in your set.

*One note: you can actually do HIT training as endurance training, since rest is fairly short and you go all the way to failure. When I use HIT for endurance training, I usually accompany it with an extended period of cardio immediately afterward.

2. So, when you're doing a typical "cardio" exercise, how does "decrease rest and decrease intensity" apply? Well, basically, rest decreases to zero. No full rest until you're done with your run (or swim or bike or what-have-you). But you need to couple that with lower intensity.

If you recall our "examen" at the beginning, your "maximum heart rate" is usually calculated as 220 bpm minus your age.

A favorite running guru of mine, Dr. Phil Maffetone (whose stuff you should check out if you're serious about gaining big endurance… ultramarathon, Ironman, stuff like that), suggests the "180 Formula" when it comes to burning fat and training endurance. Basically, you take the max heart-rate formula, but instead of 220, you subtract from 180. So if you're 30 years old, your ideal fat burning/endurance training heart rate is 150. You also modify this slightly if you haven't regularly exercised much before or are recovering from major illness (subtract another 10 bpm), if you're recovering from minor injury or have regular sinus or respiratory issues (subtract 5 bpm). On the other hand, if you're an amazing athlete with no issues, you can add 5–10 bpm. Then you train in a range with that result as the upper limit.

Okay, so, for example, I'm a fairly seasoned athlete, but I have chronic allergies and sinus infections, so while my age puts me right at about 150, I have to subtract another 5 bpm. So, I'll train in a range where I keep my heart rate between 135–145, and just try to do that for 45–90 minutes, whether I'm running, cycling, hiking, etc.

Ways to Train Endurance

So, now that we know the concepts to keep in mind during endurance training, let's look at some of the best ways to train it. We'll separate it briefly into two parts: strength and cardio.

I. STRENGTH

A. DON'T DO OLYMPIC-STYLE LIFTS

1. Wait a minute! Wasn't I saying just chapters ago how much I LOOOOOOOVE powerlifting and Olympic lifts and just wanted to MARRY THEM? Well, yes, kind of… but both of them are predicated on big compound movements, usually utilizing momentum, and stopping before failure. With endurance training, we'll be flirting with failure frequently, so if we're doing big, momentum-based movements, we're also flirting with disaster, injurywise. As a quick sidebar, this can be a major issue in the way some people do CrossFit-type workouts. Doing dozens of snatches, push presses, etc., isn't safe without careful, individual, professional supervision. Don't mess with it when training endurance.

B. OKAY, SOME POWERLIFTING MOVES CAN BE FINE

1. While I recommend you avoid Olympic lifts and others with a major momentum component, some powerlifting exercises are fine. Just do them in a controlled fashion at a higher rep range, or at least a slower rep range. Be very conscientious not to sacrifice form to get an "extra rep." I will sometimes (but rarely) do sets of 20 dead lifts or squats while being careful never to sacrifice form. If I think I can't get another rep, I will stop right then and there.

C. IN GENERAL, GO SLOW

1. One of the keys to endurance training is keeping your muscle under tension over a longer period of time. This is one of the reasons you can do HIT training for endurance as well. At minimum, you want to keep the muscle under tension for at least 1 minute and up to 2–3 minutes. So, with HIT, if you're doing 2–4

second contractions, and 4 second negatives, you only need to complete 7–10 reps to be consistently working for 1 minute. The other reason to go slow is to make sure you're not trying to operate at too high a heart rate for too long. When you're doing long strength sets, your heart rate will go up beyond that 180-minus-your-age range we're looking for, but it will come back down. If it's staying high after your rest period, lengthen the rest a little, and maybe shorten your exertion period. Like I said, a 2:1 ratio is fine. You don't have to be doing 3 minute sets with 1 minute rests… at least not until you're ready for it!

D. OUTDOOR AND BODYWEIGHT TRAINING

1. One of the best ways to train endurance is to take it outside. I'll cover trail running too, but outdoor training restricts you to what you can take with you. This can be super helpful in endurance training. If you want to practice hiking with added weight, for instance, you aren't going to be able to lug 250 pounds around with you. The sandbag I bring with me is about 60 pounds, and my tire is about 80 pounds. I already heave a heavy sigh any time I have to load them up.

2. While there are bodyweight exercises that are high intensity, like pistol squats and L-sit pull-ups, most exercises are sustainable for a higher rep range and longer duration. Think push-ups, air squats, crunches, planks, even jump squats or box jumps. Mix these into your training to make sure you're training muscular endurance as well as cardiovascular endurance.

II. CARDIOVASCULAR ENDURANCE

A. The other major part of the endurance equation is cardiovascular endurance. While doing strength training with limited rest and longer sets will keep your heart rate in an "endurance training zone" for a significant period of time, to really achieve all-around fitness you will want to train your body to maintain a lower heart rate, drain lactic-acid buildup, and benefit from all the other good stuff that comes with exerting yourself for a longer period of time.

If you're just beginning to incorporate endurance training into your fitness, doing one long session of around 90 minutes once a month should be sufficient. If you're training for a particular event, or maybe are going to be traveling and want to do a more aggressive hike somewhere, incorporating longer sessions 1–2 times a week generally becomes a good plan.

What kind of training should you do? Usually something that at least approximates the effort you're training for. If you're training for a long hike, find a hike. If you're training for a swim/bike duathlon, swim one week and bike the next. If you're training for an obstacle race, run/jog/hike trails and hills.

B. Endurance interval training serves as a way to mix up your cardio, and if you do decide to train for specific events, whether just for fun or for actual competition. Training endurance intervals helps your body get used to exerting different levels of effort for longer periods of time, which enables you to better regulate heart rate and active recovery. A lot of people will talk about different cardio "zones," which can be helpful as you get more into training. An easy rule of thumb for intervals is this: your average heart rate should fall into the endurance heart rate. So, if your endurance heart rate is 140 bpm, and you hit a hill climb that pushes you up to 160 bpm for 2 minutes, do 2 minutes of effort at 120 bpm to average it out. This happens for me all the time while trail running for obstacle racing. If there's a significant hill either up or down, it'll pull my heart rate up, so I then take it easier on the other side of that to make up for it.

C. One quick note on endurance training: my dad always told me "make sure you have the right tool for the job." When you're training endurance, this becomes very important. If you take 50,000 steps in a shoe that's wrong for you, it will negatively affect you. If you pedal 30,000 times on a bike that's poorly adjusted for you, it will negatively affect you. So, make sure to talk with someone knowledgeable about equipment in the field of whatever type of endurance training you'll be doing.

There will certainly be expensive options, but usually there are also good budget options that are totally sufficient. I've bought multiple pairs of my favorite obstacle racing shoes, and they've never cost me more than sixty dollars. Some pieces of equipment are more expensive, but usually someone knowledgeable can guide you to a solution that protects both your body and your budget.

III. SPIRITUAL ENDURANCE

A. OIU. While this might look like I simply made a mistake trying to write out an IOU, it actually stands for "Offer It Up." It simply means that when we suffer, in small ways or in large, for short or long periods of time, instead of cursing our suffering, being resentful, or complaining to anyone who will listen, we prayerfully ask God to take our sufferings, unite them with the suffering of Christ, and use them for our good and the good of others.

As Saint Paul says in Colossians 1:24, "Now I rejoice in my sufferings for your sake, and in my flesh I complete what is lacking in Christ's afflictions for the sake of his body, that is, the church." It may sound a little ethereal, but we can put it into practical terms if we look at the suffering of parents with their children. Parents cut into their own time, their money, and their outside priorities to dedicate these things to their children, out of love.

In a similar way, when we suffer, we can choose to treat our suffering not as a burden, but as something that we willingly endure for our betterment, and the benefit of others. So, when you suffer (whether it's something you choose or that just happens to you), ask God to help you embrace it, endure it, and use it to transform you and those you love.

B. Silence is golden. Praying is great. Praying for a long time can be great, too. But you know what's really great, and extremely difficult to do for a long time? Simply sitting in silence with God. I'll get much more into this in our workout portion in Part III, but one of the most valuable things you can do in your spiritual life is to set aside distraction and take a little time to sit in silence and give God the space to speak to you. Trust me, if you haven't done it before, it takes endurance!

For me, even three minutes can feel like a long time. I always want to be doing something, and silence rarely feels like doing anything. But listening, really just listening, is so important and absolutely integral to any relationship. So, always carve out time to listen to God, even when (or especially when) it feels like an endurance event.

Training endurance acclimates us to diving into longer periods of suffering in which we may have few other options than just enduring. But again, whether it's enduring one more obstacle in a race, or one more obstacle in our personal lives, take the opportunity and the challenge to offer it up and, hard as it may be, "rejoice" in it.

CHAPTER NINE
Flexibility

"Do not accept anything as the truth if it lacks love. And do not accept anything as love which lacks truth."

— Saint Teresa Benedicta of the Cross, Edith Stein

To paint with a slightly broad spiritual brush, it's common for men to hold onto truth at the expense of love and compassion, and for women to hold onto love deprived of truth. There's an over-rigidity on one side, and an overindulgence on the other. If I may point out the obvious here, that wreaks havoc on our lives and relationships.

Balance is everything. Too often we fall into the trap of latching onto one good or one truth at the expense of another, instead of living out a full, well-rounded life, philosophy, and faith. Quoting G. K. Chesterton again: "The virtues have gone mad because they have been isolated from each other and are wandering alone. Thus some scientists care for truth; and their truth is pitiless. Thus some humanitarians only care for pity; and their pity (I am sorry to say) is often untruthful."

So much of life is built on what appears to be paradoxical, a seeming contradiction that actually proves to be two truths held in harmonious tension. We are body and soul; we are called to be (like our God) both just and merciful; we are creatures given the breath of the Creator; Jesus Christ is God become human; he was born of a virgin; and died as the sinless lamb "made sin itself" to save us from sin. We Christians profess these things as true and good, but frequently have trouble letting them direct our lives.

How does this apply to physical fitness? Well, proper flexibility gives us the ability to stay healthy and fit our whole life. It prevents injury and improves muscular function. Yet, it often remains overlooked by men and overprized by women. Men can tend to be too focused on strength, thinking that stretching and flexibility are somehow a waste of time, or makes them weak. Women can focus so much on flexibility that they end up getting injured through hypermobility.

Building a healthy and balanced degree of flexibility and functional movement, then, informs both our physical and spiritual fitness.

Let's get into it.

Why Is Flexibility Important?

I think just about everyone alive has been told some philosophical parable about the strength of an oak versus the pliability of grass. The oak's proud of its strength and rude to the grass. Then a storm comes and the oak is reduced to kindling while the grass bends and gets the last laugh. Anthropomorphism and mixed metaphors aside, there are some real truths here.

When you exert yourself, you create microtears in your muscle. Without proper warm-up beforehand and proper stretching afterward, your muscles get bound up and have difficulty repairing. That can slow your progress, pull bones out of place, and push you into a cycle of injury, major strains, sprains, and tears. Heck, without a healthy degree of flexibility, you can injure yourself more easily just by sleeping, getting up from a chair, missing a step, or other minor issues, and take a long time to heal! But wait, didn't I also say being too flexible can also lead to injury? Why, yes, I did. So, let's get specific on how to find flexibility that increases health and function.

What Is a Proper Level of Flexibility?

There are two answers to this, a short one and a long one, and to my mind, the short answer's actually the more satisfying, if not the more specific. Short answer: You are at a proper level of flexibility when you can perform all the regular movements of your life, work, and leisure with economy and without pain or strain.

I'll be honest: by the short answer's standard, I'm not currently as flexible as I ought to be. For instance, I often experience a mild level of difficulty and tension (translation: pain) in my core and hamstrings when putting on socks and shoes. Do I have long femurs (thigh bones) which add to that difficulty? Yes. But that just means I need to work the flexibility of my legs and back more to compensate, not use it as an excuse. When I reach for my seat belt in my car, I sometimes use my left arm to push my right arm further to grab it. That means I'm not flexible enough in my left shoulder to grab it and pass it to my right hand. I can't reach all the way with my right hand unassisted. I'd have more economy of movement with more flexibility.

What about the question of strain? Well, this one usually applies more to women. When there's flexibility without corresponding strength, a muscle gets stretched further than it should. I had a friend who injured her wrist carrying trays in a restaurant, because as she carried the tray with her wrist at a reverse 90-degree angle, her forearm wasn't strong enough to prevent it from moving past that, but her wrist was flexible enough that the angle kept getting smaller. This led to significant pain down the road, even though there wasn't any at the time. Another friend of mine popped a tendon merely by standing up from a seated position on a low seat with her legs and feet flexed far underneath her. Because she was flexible, she got into a position that she didn't have the strength to get out of safely. So, having significantly more flexibility than strength isn't proper flexibility either!

Okay, so that's the short answer, made longer by a couple of examples. The long answer is a more specific, but less universal, checklist. Since it's less universal, you'll generally want to check these standards with a medical professional to make sure they fit your actual capabilities. These are standards you want to get to eventually, not force yourself to reach today. Remember, if you're straining, in significant or stabbing pain, or jerking around, you're doing flexibility wrong. Here's the checklist:

1. LEGS

a) On a two-leg or single-leg floor touch, you should be able to touch your toes without pain or strain. If you're flexible enough that you are folding in half without strain, be sure you have corresponding leg and core strength to support that flexibility.

b) On a quad stretch, you should be able to stand upright and have your heel touch your butt without pain or strain. (Photo 239, Page 190)

c) On a groin stretch, you should have the capability to pull your heels all the way to your groin if you're a woman, and at least within 8–12 inches of your groin if you're a man. Why the difference here? Men and women generally have structurally different levels of hip flexibility... the reason: babies.

d) On a calf stretch, the leg being stretched should be at a 45-degree angle, with the heel on the ground without discomfort. (Photo 240, Page 190)

2. BACK

a) If you bend at the waist, you should be able to get to a 90-degree angle with a flat or only minimally rounded back. If it's significantly rounded, you need more flexibility.

b) When you do a trunk twist, you should be able to open your body up almost to fully sideways on both sides.

3. CHEST AND SHOULDERS

a) On a one-arm chest stretch, you should be able to stand up straight with your chest out and have your arm parallel or nearly parallel to the floor, and at almost a 90-degree angle to your body. If you can go past that while parallel to the floor, you need to be careful to make sure you have sufficient strength to support that extra flexibility, because a straight arm isn't really made to go much further.

b) On the back-scratch test, your fingers should at least touch on both sides. If you can hold fingertips with yourself, that's fine. If you can grab your wrists, the admonition about having corresponding strength applies.

c) While doing a one-arm shoulder stretch, you should be able to stretch a straight arm nearly flat against your body.

4. ARMS

a) The same flexibility guidelines apply to a one-arm bicep stretch as a one-arm chest stretch.

b) The back-scratch test for shoulders can also test your triceps. Or do a one-arm tricep stretch: your upper arm of the stretched arm should be in line with your body, and your body upright. Significantly past that risks injury.

c) With your forearms and wrists, your hand should be able to easily rest at 90 degrees forward or backward without any assistance, and it's fine if you can stretch it a little past that. If you can lie your hand flat against your wrist on either side without much effort, you need to be sure to have strong forearms to protect your wrist.

Okay, that's the long answer to "what is proper flexibility?" Now we need to talk about how to train it.

How to Train Flexibility

I like to measure flexibility across three dimensions: ballistic, isometric, and static. Ballistic is flexibility while moving (like doing hurdles, or the "hug" stretch found in the exercise guide). Isometric is the flexibility and strength needed to hold a body position under effort (like having your shoulders in a proper position during a handstand). Static refers to when you simply hold a stretched position for the purpose of stretching the muscle (like any of the stretch tests, or any time you're directed to "hold" a stretch).

My wife (who was a kinesiology major, personal trainer, and semipro athlete) says, "Ballistic before, static after." Basically, you should get muscles and joints moving before you do a workout. In other words, use ballistic stretches and warm-ups to, well, warm-up. Don't do static stretches prior to a workout; you can easily overstretch or weaken a muscle and injure yourself. Chances are it's not warm and not ready to be manually stretched. During a workout, you may do exercises that require isometric strength. Always be sure you're using proper form. After you are done working your muscles, use static stretching to cool down, remove the lactic-acid buildup, and finish up the workout.

On days when you're working out, you should do 5–10 minutes of warm-up, and 5–10 minutes of cool down. On days when you're not working out, you should still do 5–10 minutes of ballistic stretching, followed by 5–10 minutes of static stretching. The form that takes will vary daily, depending on what muscles you've been training, what kinds of exercise and leisure you've been pursuing, what body positions your daily life finds you in, etc. Regardless of the variables, give yourself a total of 10–20 minutes of stretching (half ballistic and half static) every day. That's how to train flexibility, and that's what you'll see in our workouts.

Finally, what about spiritual flexibility? How do you avoid the "lactic-acid buildup" of legalism and self-righteousness on one side and the "ligament strain" of a lack of discipline and truth? Good question. Here again, we'll dive more deeply into this in our workouts (yes, there's a spirituality portion). But the principle is the same: keep moving and stretching while building corresponding strength.

Open yourself up to God in silence and contemplative prayer while also committing to disciplines like fasting, attending an extra Mass one day a week, and so on. Study the Faith, but do it prayerfully. Search out and practice a spirituality that's uncomfortable for you. That might mean praying a Rosary if you're a spontaneous praying kind of person, or dipping a toe into Catholic mysticism and contemplation if you tend to use a lot of verbal prayers. One way that directly correlates to flexibility training that I like goes like this: arrive early to Mass (What? I know, how dare I even suggest that?), spend 5–10 minutes reading through the readings and Gospel for the day, and meditate on them. Be "present" for Mass. Then spend 10–20 minutes just sitting in the church afterward, with perhaps some praying, but mostly silence, to be with God who's present in the tabernacle, and within you. Do that consistently and you'll be surprised how much it irons out the kinks in your spiritual life!

CHAPTER TEN
"The Training Trinity" (Exercise, Rest, and Nutrition)

"We acknowledge the Trinity, holy and perfect, to consist of the Father, the Son and the Holy Spirit. In this Trinity there is no intrusion of any alien element or of anything from outside, nor is the Trinity a blend of creative and created being. It is a wholly creative and energizing reality, self-consistent and undivided in its active power, for the Father makes all things through the Word and in the Holy Spirit, and in this way the unity of the holy Trinity is preserved."

— Saint Athanasius the Great

As I wrote in Chapter Four, the *Catechism* says that the Trinity is "the central mystery of Christian faith and life" (234). We see reflections of the Trinity all around us. We see it in the choices we make for good or ill, because we have the capability to know, to love, and to decide. We see it in our human nature, that we are a unity of body, mind, and soul. And while it would be blasphemous to claim that "The Training Trinity" is anywhere near as important (it definitely isn't), it too is a kind of central mystery which leads to health and fitness.

Exercise, rest, and nutrition simply do not work in isolation. They are all essential, not as parts, but as one whole. They energize your life, your work, everything you do. Exercise without either proper nutrition or rest will only break down your muscles and body. Rest divided from either nutrition or exercise will leave you fat or atrophied. Proper nutrition without exercise still leads to a host of health problems. And without rest, you simply wear your body out. So, in this section, we'll talk about how to properly balance exercise, rest, and nutrition for a more active, creative, and energized life!

Exercise

I know we've talked a lot about exercise so far, so I won't belabor any points here. It's easy, however, to make the mistake of treating exercise as if it's the only thing that matters — as though training harder or more often will always be a benefit. Perhaps that's because exercise is tangible. We can feel the work, see the sweat, experience the intensity of a workout well-done. By contrast, rest and nutrition can be harder to understand in a tangible way. We don't always feel a victory when we exercise the discipline of getting to bed on time, or eating the right balance of macronutrients for our goals. At least, I don't feel the same level of excitement between lifting a new personal record and eating more turkey instead of pecan pie at Thanksgiving.

The same can be true in our spiritual lives: We can easily feel like we always have to be *doing* to have it count, whether it's reading and studying the Bible, praying memorized prayers, or committing ourselves to extremely difficult Lenten practices. I'm reminded of a verse from Isaiah: "This people draw near with their mouth / and honor me with their lips, / while their hearts are far from me" (Is 29:13). I for one, definitely feel accomplishment when I complete a Rosary… which means I'm probably forgetting the fact that the point of the Rosary is meditation and relationship. Just like in exercise, we're looking for intensity, not merely activity.

The fact is that sometimes (actually quite frequently), God does the greatest works where we don't immediately perceive it. I think of 1 Kings 19:11–13, where the Lord passes by Elijah who is taking shelter in a cave: "And behold, the LORD passed by, and a great and strong wind rent the mountains, and broke in pieces the rocks before the LORD, but the LORD was not in the wind; and after the wind an earthquake, but the LORD was not in the earthquake; and after the earthquake a fire, but the LORD was not in the fire; and after the fire a still small voice." That is the voice of God, and it guides him to his next big task.

In our lives, we frequently look for big signs and massive change. But whether we're talking about signs and change in our souls or in our bodies, we miss the important lesson that God is consistently calling us to faith. Jesus says, "An evil and adulterous generation seeks for a sign" (Mt 16:4). However, he frequently gives us the opportunity to trust, to have faith: "Now faith is the assurance of things hoped for, the conviction of things not seen" (Heb 11:1).

So, whether it's prayer, exercise, rest, or nutrition, we may experience the feeling that our work isn't doing anything, that we don't see any change. But God has made your heart, your mind, your body, and your soul to respond to the good things you do. That paves the way for his grace, and that's when change occurs.

If you find yourself stuck on exercise, or don't feel any progress, check your rest and nutrition, and if they are where they need to be, then just trust the process. If you are eating properly, but it's hard and you don't see change, you may be tempted to say, "What's the point?" Trust me, God is working unseen in your body as he is in your soul. Keep offering your challenges to him. Sometimes change is obvious and happens quickly. But more often, it takes patience, diligence, and self-control over time to achieve your goals.

You can see complete transformation in your body in 90 days, and I believe it's possible to see that in your soul, too. But you absolutely won't if you give up every couple of days. Start small, do what you can, and trust that your daily exercise is tilling the soil for the growth that God's grace will provide.

Rest

I think it was during college that I first recognized a horrible, destructive, misguided game people play that I like to call "What's Sleep?" The rules are simple: if you sleep, you lose. Everyone loses eventually, but there are those elite players who really give a good go of it by eking out only two to five hours of sleep each night. I theorize that we (perhaps especially in America) associate productivity with busyness and rest with laziness. This simply isn't true. Remember that even God rested on the seventh day and gave us the Sabbath for the same purpose. This isn't just a nice story to help the weak and slothful among us justify themselves. It's a necessary part of life! One of my favorite prayers is part of night prayer from the Liturgy of the Hours, where it says, "May the Lord grant us a restful night and a peaceful death." The psalmist says in Psalm 4:9, "In peace I will both lie down and sleep; for thou alone, O LORD, makest me dwell in safety."

Proper rest not only brings us closer to God and lets us exercise trust in him (the saints often speak of prayer as "resting in God"), but, in fact, rest is the very thing God created to allow us to heal and develop.

What do I mean by that? Well, if we're using our bodies properly, we push ourselves to grow and change. The only time we actually grow and change, however, is when we're resting. If you're trying to reach or maintain a level of fitness, you push your body past what it's accustomed to doing. Then when you rest, it has the opportunity to repair and create a new status quo. If you don't rest properly, you just wear your body out. Imagine driving cross country without stopping. No fill-ups, no oil changes, no bathroom breaks. Neither you nor your car would make it very far. And you might have caused irreparable damage in the process.

The same holds true for proper rest and recovery. Most human beings need about seven-and-a-half hours of sleep a night: some need a little more, very few need a little less. But you don't win any prizes for grinding by on three hours a night! Unless you consider heart disease, depression, premature aging, obesity, hormone imbalance, Alzheimer's, and early death to be "prizes." There's a big health gap even between people who get six hours of sleep rather than seven-and-a-half. Worse still, studies show that people who regularly sleep six hours think that they've "adapted" to it, but when tested on mental alertness and performance, they perform worse.

On a spiritual level, getting less than seven-and-a-half hours of sleep a night can make you significantly more susceptible to sin. It exacerbates the weakened will and dimmed intellect we've received from the Fall. When you're tired, it's harder to resist temptation — whether it's lust, gluttony, anger and irritability, greed... the list goes on. So, to take proper care of your whole person, sleep seven-and-a-half hours a night. Okay, if you have a new baby in the house, you may need to temporarily adjust that mandate. But other excuses, particularly any having to do with productivity ("I need to study more!" "I need to get extra work done!" "I just gotta get my cardio in!"), do not fly. Why? Remember, your actual level of productivity takes a nose dive when you lose sleep. Sleep the extra hour. You'll get your studying, work, or exercise done more effectively and efficiently if you do, and it will be plenty sufficient to make up for the "lost time."

Now, on the other side of the equation, if you find yourself wasting away the day by sleeping 10–12 hours, you'll need to rein that in! I'm not trying to promote sloth here, just an appropriate level of rest. If you struggle with oversleeping, try going to bed at a set time every night, and earlier rather than later. Our bodies are primarily designed to be awake when the sun is up and asleep when the sun is down. Obviously, with the way we humans have set up our work/school/life hours, that can be a challenge, particularly when it's a time of year that daylight lasts only 10 hours or so! But, as a rule of thumb, a consistent schedule of getting to bed by 9–10 p.m. and waking up at 5–6 a.m. has cured many an oversleeper.

So that covers our main issues with sleep. But what about other forms of proper physical rest, relaxation, recuperation, etc.? When is it good to just, you know, veg out on the couch for half a day while binge-watching your favorite show (and probably binge-eating in the process)? Unfortunately, that's just plain never a good idea. One of the most physically taxing things I ever did was go to a theater and watch the three *Lord of the Rings* movies (extended editions), back-to-back-to-back in a 13-hour movie marathon. By the end of it, my whole body hurt. I felt weary and burned out through inactivity.

Outside of sleep, we operate best when we are engaged in easy activity most of the day, moderate activity some of the day, and intense activity in several intervals through the week. You'll see this reflected in our workouts. I'll have you working hard for relatively short periods, 3–5 times a week. Then you rest 2–3 times a week. But even on "rest days," you should be engaging in easy to moderate activity: walking, going up and down stairs, stretching, hiking, playing a sport for fun, and so on. If you work a job that keeps you sitting all day, I really encourage you to find even just 2–3 minutes an hour to get up, do squats, jumping jacks, or Burpees, and stretch a little. Don't spend all day sitting. Your body isn't made for that.

What about the question of recuperation that I promised to answer? "You don't expect me to exercise when I'm sick, right?" Should you give up on praying when you're tired or experiencing temptation? In case there's any confusion, the answer to that slightly rhetorical question is certainly "no." Exercise releases super-beneficial endorphins and other hormones that can actually help you get well sooner, so you don't have to quit exercising when you're sick. That said, if you are sick, it's always important to seek proper medical attention. Like proper rest, that's not a "weak" thing to do. Also, there are some symptoms that will certainly adjust what you're doing. Let's look at them:

- If your symptoms are "neck up," no change needed. So, if you've got a sore throat, runny nose, allergy attack, or anything like that, take the medicine you need to treat your symptoms and do your workout. Do add extra fluid intake and extra sleep to help your body heal, though.
- When it comes to coughing, moderate your activity level. I had severe bronchitis as a child and it has forever altered the way my lungs respond to irritation. Once I start coughing, I won't stop until I completely stop moving. So when I have a cough, I may choose to do a slow uphill walk or easy hike, or an easier weightlifting routine where I'm only working smaller muscle groups, like arms. If I try to do squats, fast running, etc., I'm forcing my lungs to take in more air more rapidly than they want to without freaking out. So, go easier, but don't avoid exercise or activity entirely. The same admonition about increased water and sleep applies here as above.
- Stomach illnesses, like vomiting, sudden and unexpected bowel stuff, etc., serve as the exception to the rule. Don't exercise when you're sick with these. Just sleep, rest, and get better. Your body will usually kick these symptoms within a couple of days anyhow, so exercise certainly isn't going to speed recovery here.

All right, so that covers sleep, rest, recovery, and recuperation. Now, as awkward a segue as it might be to go from talking about vomiting to talking about eating… that's what we're going to do. On to nutrition!

Nutrition

Along with proper rest, nutrition is the other component that contributes to proper recovery. Imagine the whole physical fitness process as putting an addition on your house. The exercise knocks down the old walls, but it's proper nutrition that rebuilds the house bigger and better.

Like I mentioned when talking about flexibility and when talking about rest, exercise pushes us past what we're used to doing. This creates microtears in your muscles, forcing your body to repair and rebuild to deal with that stimulus. This is how the process works for every single component of fitness. However, if you don't give yourself the time to rebuild (rest), or if you neglect giving it the actual raw materials to rebuild (nutrition), exercise will just break you down.

On the other hand, if you give your body too much in the way of raw materials, it will (to abuse our building metaphor a little more) put that in storage… generally as fat. Proper nutrition, a proper intake of both macronutrients (protein, carbohydrate, and fat) and micronutrients (vitamins and minerals), comprises an integral part of recovery and ongoing health.

What in the supernatural parallels the natural? Well, in John 6:35, Jesus says, "I am the bread of life; he who comes to me shall not hunger, and he who believes in me shall never thirst." Catholics believe that this goes a lot further than simple metaphor, that God reveals a truth to the truism "you are what you eat." Reading the Bible (which we might equate to exercise) and praying (which can be thought of as "resting in God") are great and essential, but without the sacraments — and the Eucharist in particular — "you have no life in you" (Jn 6:53). Our lives are incomplete without truly being fed by God, becoming one with him in holy Communion.

There's another spiritual connection that ties into the physical: What we eat everyday *does* demonstrate how we feel about this temple of the Holy Spirit that God has given us. If Jesus came to dinner, you wouldn't serve him Twinkies and chips (at least I hope you wouldn't). Well, "Do you not know that you are God's temple and that God's Spirit dwells in you?" (1 Cor 3:16). Treat the temple of your body with the dignity it deserves when considering what you consistently put in it. The choices you make physically reveal a deeper spiritual reality.

Okay, we've got a lot of ground to cover to hit the basics, so this will be a long section… but I encourage you to go beyond the basics. There are plenty of great books on nutrition, and I recommend you find and read a few of those. I'm not talking about books on fad diets, but on proper nutrition. This section is a primer course; as in every aspect of your life, it behooves you to constantly keep learning, striving, and growing!

I. CALORIES

A. WHAT ARE CALORIES?

1. We'll get to macronutrients in a second — they're the nutrients that actually provide calories — but let's talk about what calories are and how to use them. Strictly speaking, what we commonly call calories are technically kilocalories, a measurement of energy: 1 calorie contains enough energy to raise 1 gram of water by 1 degree Celsius, while 1 kilocalorie contains enough energy to raise 1 kilogram of water by 1 degree Celsius. We human beings use thousands of kilocalories daily. However, since we hate stumbling over long words, we commonly just call kilocalories "calories," even though that's technically totally inaccurate. (It's an inaccuracy that I'm going to go ahead and continue using, because everybody does and so it's simpler.)

So, all of that said, what's the important thing to learn? Calories are energy. They're not good or bad, they just are what they are. Now, to get far more or far fewer than you need would be bad, because it causes health risks, so let's look at that. Just remember, in and of themselves, calories are not good or bad. So don't freak out if something has a lot of calories… just figure out whether or not that fits into your current nutrition needs and move on.

B. CALORIE SURPLUS, CALORIE DEFICIT, AND BASAL METABOLIC RATE

1. What are these?

a) When we talk about calorie surplus and calorie deficit, we're talking about whether the amount of calories you're taking in exceeds the amount your body requires for basic function and daily activity, or whether that amount falls short. Since your daily activity levels fluctuate, the amount of calories necessary to cover those changes. Once you reach adulthood though, the amount of calories required for basic function tends to stay fairly consistent, although it generally decreases over time.

But there are no major fluctuations in it like there are in activity levels. The amount of calories required for your body to maintain basic functions is called your basal metabolic rate (BMR). Because there aren't major fluctuations, it's actually pretty simple to calculate! But while the equation is simple, it's not exactly easy, so honestly, just do an Internet search for "calculate basal metabolic rate," and you'll find what you need. It should let you enter height, weight, age, sex, and activity level. Well, technically as soon as you enter your activity level, it's really giving you a measure of your resting metabolic rate (RMR), but that's more what we're looking for anyway.

The difference is that BMR is calculating simply the calories that it takes to keep you alive, and RMR is calculating those calories plus the calories needed for basic activities like chewing, standing up and sitting down, brushing your teeth, etc. One thing to note about BMR and RMR: fat is energy storage, muscle is a consumer of energy. So the more muscle you have, the more energy (calories) your body will consume on a regular basis… meaning a higher BMR and RMR. Why does all that matter? Oh, look, that's the heading of the next section!

2. WHY DOES ALL THAT MATTER?

a) At the simplest level, if you are regularly in calorie surplus (more calories than your BMR/RMR plus the calories required for your exercise and other activities), you will gain weight. If you are regularly in calorie deficit (fewer calories than your BMR/RMR plus the calories required for your exercise and other activities), you will lose weight. Basically, if your body has extra energy (calories), it will find a way to use it (by building muscle) or store it (as body fat). If your body needs more energy, it will find stored calories on you somewhere and use those (the key is to make it burn fat and not muscle). How do we figure all that out? Well, through a proper understanding and use of macronutrients.

II. MACRONUTRIENTS
A. WHAT ARE MACRONUTRIENTS?

1. To understand how your body works at a basic level, you need to have some understanding of macronutrients. These are the major types of nutrients that all foods contain, and the kinds of nutrients that provide calories. As I mentioned, that's protein, carbohydrate, and fat.

Now despite what the fad diet/lifestyle hack/neopagan spiritualist philosophy might have told you, your body actually needs *all* of them. It's true that our bodies are incredible at improvising in times of necessity, as some of these trendy diets force them to do, but a balanced and sustainable life involves the proper use of each of the macronutrients. As a fun exercise, take a week to "track your macros." See how many grams of protein, carbohydrate, and fat you're consuming. Even before reading this section, you might be surprised with what you find. And after reading this section, you'll have a lot clearer idea of what they all mean. Read your labels, jot it down, and if you get stuck, there are lots of macro-tracking apps that have information that you might not have, so check those out. But what do each of the macronutrients do, and how do we consume them in the proper proportions? Let's take a look.

B. FAT

1. Fat may still be the reigning champion of misunderstood macronutrients, although in recent years, carbohydrate has started to give it a run for its money. Generally, we tend to think of fat that we consume having a direct correlation to fat on us (which seems to make us go, "ew, gross!"). As with most things in life, there's a half-truth to this… but also as with most things, the devil's in the half-truth.

As we discussed, if you eat in a calorie surplus, you will gain weight. Now, if you eat a lot of fat, you consume a lot of calories… making it far easier to eat in a calorie surplus. The reason is because while one gram of carbohydrate or protein has 4 calories, one gram of fat has 9 calories. If you were to consume exactly the same amount of fat as you did either protein or carbohydrate, you would have consumed more than twice as many calories. So the half-truth is that fat quickly packs on calories, which, if that leads to a calorie surplus, can definitely add fat to you. However, you always need to consume at least some fat. Your body needs fat to run properly, and cannot produce certain kinds of fats. Essential fats protect our vital organs, aid protein use, and start chemical reactions that keep our major body systems (nervous system, immune system, reproductive system) functioning properly.

Nevertheless, we don't generally need most of the kinds or quantity of fat that we consume in say, fast food, or by adding fats to every meal. Some people think, "Well, butter's bad, but margarine/olive oil/coconut oil/fill-in-your-trendy-fat-of-choice is good for you. Load me up!" In a very basic sense, it's true that some sources of fat are "cleaner," or contain more essential fatty acids, than other sources, but they still contain double the calories of other macronutrients. So, most people don't need to try hard to consume a sufficient amount of fat. When I consume fat, I try to consume it from less-processed sources, and do not add it to anything I consume. What do I mean by that? I don't use butter, olive oil, or sour cream as a topping. I will sometimes use a teaspoon or so of fat in my cooking, while sautéing, roasting, etc., just to prevent stuff from burning. But adding fat for flavor? Almost never. Why? Because I nearly always get plenty of fat from the actual foods I'm consuming. I'll have a couple of eggs at breakfast, and handful or two of nuts during the day. Maybe chicken thighs and a little avocado at lunch, and lean beef at dinner. Across the day then, I'm probably getting 60–75 grams of fat, which is more than sufficient for my body's needs, and provides somewhere between 540–675 calories.

There are some people who undertake ketogenic diets, where they force their body into a state of ketosis (using fat as the primary source of energy, rather than carbohydrate) by consuming almost no carbohydrate, moderate amounts of protein, and getting most of their calories through consuming fat. That's a specialized diet, I've used it several times in my life, and don't have a problem with it. But (and this is a *big* caveat), if you're going to do it, you really need to understand it. WAY too many people think: "Eat lots of fat? Got it. Bacon, eggs, steak, hamburgers, let's go!" They end up skyrocketing the amount of calories consumed and cause more health problems. So, I'll repeat: If you're going to take on a ketogenic diet, you really need to understand it. We don't have the space here to go into the details of it, but there are plenty of resources out there to understand it. If you want to try it, research it first!

C. CARBOHYDRATE

1. Like I said earlier, carbohydrate is currently vying to overtake fat for the top spot in "most misunderstood macronutrients." We've turned a corner in America especially, where we've stopped fearing a high-fat diet and now have a knee-jerk aversion to "carbs." But most people don't know why.

Let's look at the truth again here: our bodies are, generally speaking, made to use carbohydrate as our primary energy source. We are not naturally ketogenic (see above), except in time of great necessity, when there is no regularly available source of carbohydrate, and so our body switches its process. Another important thing to remember: many foods dense in micronutrients (which we'll address shortly) contain carbohydrate. So, you don't absolutely, unequivocally need carbohydrate (we can function in a ketogenic state), but your body's "factory settings" certainly prefer it!

Where does the problem lie? Eating carbohydrate to a calorie surplus from micronutrient-poor sources! We load ourselves up on sugars, flours, breads, potatoes, and so on — high carbohydrate foods with almost no micronutrients. What should we do? Eat a sufficient amount of carbohydrate to supply our basic energy needs as part of a balanced diet, and choose sources that provide lots of micronutrients. That primarily means green vegetables, beans, sweet potato, whole grains still in their grain state — for example, quinoa, bulgur wheat, whole or cut oats, and NOT "whole grain" bread, instant oatmeal, etc.

You might notice that I haven't included fruit on this list. Why not? Well, most fruits, while they do have some micronutrients, also pack a ton of calories, and so they're not the most efficient way to get those nutrients. Honestly, the most efficient way to get nutrients is through vegetables, and we'll talk more about that in the micronutrient section. For now, suffice it to say that unless you're trying for serious and rapid weight gain, you rarely need to eat anything just for the calories, which is really all fruit has to offer over other options. The only time I tend to eat fruit is directly following a workout. I'll add a little fruit to a protein shake after a workout, because the sugar in the fruit replenishes glycogen stores and aids protein absorption immediately after intense effort. And the sugar tastes nice, too. But just because something tastes good doesn't make it good. Take fruit juices, for example. The conventional juicing process pretty much robs fruit of the best thing it has going for it, which is fiber, and it loses other micronutrients in the process as well. So by the time you're sipping your morning orange juice, you almost might as well be drinking a morning Coke. Or hummingbird nectar.

Okay, long story a little less long than it could be? Eat a sufficient amount of carbohydrate to supply your basic energy needs, and get that from micronutrient-dense sources. We'll talk about how to do that in the next section. But first, let's talk about our last macronutrient.

D. PROTEIN

1. Just because I mentioned "most misunderstood macronutrients" for both of our other two macros, I feel compelled to mention protein's standing here: least misunderstood. Almost no one says, "Protein is so bad for you, right?" Most people basically understand that it builds and maintains muscles, which we see as good. We might further love protein if we know that it's also integral in producing healthy hair, skin, nails, bones, cartilage, blood, essential hormones and enzymes.

And when it comes to the Training Trinity (oh, yeah, remember how that's what this chapter's about?), it's the only macronutrient that has an immediate and direct correlation to the repair of your muscles, because it's the only macronutrient that *can* repair your muscles. Yes, you need carbohydrate to get enough calories to get through the day, and fat to keep your major systems functioning, but as far as repair goes, protein is key.

How much protein do you need, and where should you get it from? When you're exercising regularly, you need 0.6 to 0.8 grams of protein per pound of bodyweight, just to repair. If you want to make progress, generally you need 1 to 1.2 grams per pound of bodyweight, and I've met athletes who are trying to gain muscle rapidly who will hit 1.5 to nearly 2 grams per pound of bodyweight.

What does that look like? As of this writing, I'm about 180 pounds. If I want to continue to progress, I should take in 180–216 grams of protein daily. That's actually a pretty high amount. It equates to about 30 eggs, or 3 steaks, or almost a whole chicken. So, you need to be sure you're getting it from sources that don't impede your other macronutrient goals. For instance, if I get 200 grams of protein from bacon, I'm going to have about 1,000 more calories from fat than I want. If I decide to get 200 grams of protein from rice and beans, I'll probably explode before I'm finished consuming the total of 7,000 calories and 10 pounds of food it would take. I'll generally eat lean protein sources a couple of times a day (chicken, fish, egg whites), a fattier protein source (like beef or sometimes pork) once a day, and supplement with a protein shake (usually protein is almost the only macronutrient in there) once a day. I also usually make sure that my carbohydrate sources also have some amount of protein — for example, beans, quinoa.

Like I mentioned at the beginning of the section on macronutrients, once you track what you're taking in over the course of a week, you will find it much easier.

One final, important note on protein: When I talked about calorie deficit and calorie surplus, I said in passing that you want to be sure to burn fat and not to lose muscle when you're losing weight. So how do you do that? Two simple steps: always, always, always get at least 1 gram of protein per pound of bodyweight; and always, always, always strength train. That way, when your body is looking to burn calories that you're not providing it, it uses your fat stores rather than your muscle. Why? Because it sees that you are actively and aggressively using your muscles, and that it needs sufficient protein to repair them, it will work to get its energy elsewhere. If you slacken off on your strength training (or worse, stop it entirely and think "I just need to do cardio"), or don't get sufficient protein, your body will see your muscle as an unnecessary calorie drain (as mentioned, muscle takes more calories to sustain), and stop feeding it, leading to muscle atrophy, a slowed metabolism, reduced BMR, and higher body fat levels, not lower ones. Got it? Good.

III. MICRONUTRIENTS

A. WHAT ARE MICRONUTRIENTS AND HOW ARE THEY DIFFERENT THAN MACRONUTRIENTS?

1. Very simply, "micronutrients" means vitamins and minerals, chemical elements that your body only needs in small (micro) amounts, rather than in large (macro) amounts.

2. Unlike protein, carbohydrate, and fat (macronutrients), which we generally measure in grams, micronutrients are almost always measured in milligrams (1/1000 gram).

3. Micronutrients also don't provide calories. Now this doesn't mean you can't overdo certain micronutrients, you absolutely can. Some micronutrients that

our body needs (vitamin A, vitamin D, iron, to name a few) are highly toxic in higher doses. If you are supplementing with vitamins and minerals, please, please, please, research proper dosages so you don't end up one of the 60,000 cases of vitamin poisoning that occur in the United States each year. More on how to avoid that in a second.

B. WAIT, WHAT'S FIBER?
1. One nutrient that sometimes gets lumped in with micronutrients is fiber. Technically, it's not a micronutrient. You do need it in macro quantities. You should have approximately 14 grams of fiber for every 1,000 calories you're consuming in a day. Why do some people toss it in with micronutrients (which I guess I'm doing here)? Well, because fiber also doesn't provide calories. Your body can't digest dietary fiber, so it can't absorb any calories out of it. It can't digest it but, boy, does it try. The work of trying but being unable to digest fiber keeps your intestines strong, cleaned out, and working well. So get your fiber!

C. HOW DO YOU AVOID OVERDOSING ON MICRONUTRIENTS?
1. The simplest answer to this is that you should get almost all your micronutrients in sufficient quantities from your diet. It's pretty hard to overdose on micronutrients out of whole foods. Vitamin and mineral supplements, then, should be used as just that: supplements. They supplement what you are getting out of the food that you eat. They shouldn't attempt to replace it.

2. Research what micronutrients you are getting from your diet, and if you see the need to supplement, research what you're taking, and what quantities it is safe to have. For instance, some people will supplement with Niacin, and not realize it's the same thing as the vitamin B3 supplement they're also taking, and overdose on that. So, if you're going to supplement, make sure you take the time to develop a clear and safe game plan.

D. WHAT KIND OF FOODS PROVIDE MICRONUTRIENTS?
1. First and foremost: vegetables. I eat lots of vegetables daily, usually two different vegetables at every meal, and in fairly large quantities. Leafy greens (and generally the darker the green, the better) contain lots of great micronutrients and are also low in calories, so they don't overload you. Same with cruciferous vegetables, like broccoli, Brussel sprouts, collard greens, kale, etc.

Root vegetables like carrots and beets, while more sugary and higher in calories, provide everything from beta carotene (the precursor to vitamin A) to folate to betaine. Peppers are full of vitamins B2, B6, C, and E. Mushrooms (okay, they're a fungus, not a vegetable) have lots of B vitamins, vitamin D, a handful of minerals, and also may positively affect your immune system.

Basically, you can consume a ton of vegetables and get most of your micronutrient needs met without getting too many calories. Also, most vegetables (even organic ones) are fairly inexpensive.

Not a huge veggie fan? Pro tip: lightly sauté leafy greens (or the leafier cruciferous ones, like kale and collard greens) with a tiny bit of salt and pepper, pan sear mushrooms (salt and pepper again), roast everything else. There are great ways to season vegetables that don't add fat calories (don't dunk them in ranch dressing, cover them in butter, smother them in cheese, etc.), so you can love them as much as your body does!

2. Certain minerals are best found in animal sources. Fish is high in calcium, selenium, B12, and iodine. Beef is rich in iron, magnesium, and creatine. Chicken is filled with phosphorous and B6. Eggs contain choline, B2, and B12. So, as you're getting your protein for the day, try to eat from a variety of sources.

IV. PUTTING IT ALL TOGETHER

A. Okay, now that you know the basics of macro- and micronutrients, calories, and metabolic rate, what do you do with it? You figure out what your caloric needs are based on your BMR or RMR and your exercise, you decide whether to be in calorie deficit or surplus, and you pick a variety of foods that will meet those goals and also provide plenty of micronutrients. As far as macronutrient breakdown, your first priority is always to get sufficient protein. Unless you have researched and are implementing a ketogenic diet, fat calories should generally occupy about 25–30% of your total caloric intake, and carbohydrate can fill the remainder. Here are two quick examples I've used, one for calorie deficit, one for calorie surplus. Your needs will vary, but this is a good basic starting point.

1. EXAMPLE CALORIE DEFICIT NEEDS:
   a) BMR + activity = 2,700 calories
   b) Calorie deficit of 500 calories daily = 2,200 total calories needed
   c) Weight of 180 pounds = protein intake of 1 gram per pound = 180 grams/720 calories (approximately 33% of total calories needed)
   d) Fat calories at 25% of total calories = 550 calories, or about 61 grams of fat (remember, fat contains 9 calories per gram versus the 4 calories per gram in protein and carbohydrate)

e) Remainder of calories (2,200 minus 1,270 from protein and fat) = 930. 930/4 = 232.5 grams carbohydrate.

f) Breakdown: Protein = 180 grams (720 calories, 33% of total calories); Fat = 61 grams (550 calories, 25% of total calories); Carbohydrate = 232.5 grams (930 calories, 42% of total calories)

2. EXAMPLE CALORIE SURPLUS NEEDS:

a) BMR + activity = 2,700 calories

b) Calorie surplus of 500 calories daily = 3,200 total calories needed

c) Weight of 180 pounds = protein intake of 1.25 gram per pound (more protein because here I'm trying to gain more muscle) = 225 grams/900 calories (approximately 28% of total calories needed)

d) Fat calories at 25% of total calories = 800 calories, or about 89 grams of fat

e) Remainder of calories (3,200 minus 1,700 from protein and fat) = 1,500. 1,500/4 = 375 grams carbohydrate

f) Breakdown: Protein = 225 grams (900 calories, 28% of total calories); Fat = 61 grams (550 calories, 25% of total calories); Carbohydrate = 375 grams (1500 calories, 47% of total calories)

I know that was a lot of information. We covered all the aspects of the Training Trinity: exercise, rest, and nutrition. Now it's time to take all this knowledge you've just amassed and put it into practice. In *The Imitation of Christ*, Thomas à Kempis writes, "I had rather feel contrition than know its definition." Knowing "how to pray" does us no good unless we do it, knowing what is good does us no good unless we do it, a knowledge of self-control doesn't change us, but exercising self-control does. So, in the coming workouts, we'll live out the integration of person, body and soul, that we've been talking about. We'll let God grow our virtues and graces to imbue every part of our lives.

Set aside excuses and fears, and let's do it.

PART 3
The Workouts

A NOVENA CHALLENGE

In the life of the faithful, a novena serves as a nine-day period of prayer and petition, usually accompanied by some form of suffering. As Saint Jerome notes, "The number nine in Holy Writ is indicative of suffering and grief."

As we talked about in the Chapter Two on suffering, nearly all good things involve our dying to self and doing something difficult. However, this shouldn't scare us or frustrate us. Rather, we should look at suffering as an opportunity to be stripped of our unnecessary attachments and to become stronger as we are revealed to ourselves. As Thomas à Kempis says, "Times of trouble best discover the true worth of a man; they do not weaken him, but show his true nature."

The good news is that the suffering involved in this novena mainly comes from doing something that you're unused to… whether that's the prayer portion or the workouts. Neither the prayer nor the workouts are unduly burdensome in and of themselves. As with all novenas, take this as a time to trust in God and in the process, and get excited to take this first step to new growth.

For the prayer portion of each day's workout we'll be doing one thing that most people do rarely, and one thing that most people almost never do, including most Catholics. We'll start by expressing gratitude, picking the first three things to be grateful for that come to mind. Then we'll simply spend five minutes in silence. Don't pray Hail Marys, don't ask for anything from God, don't quiz yourself on world capitals (am I the only person who does that?), just sit as close to silence and as close to zero distractions as possible for five minutes.

You can meditate on the things you've just expressed gratitude for, but try to talk less and listen more. Set a timer so you're not checking your watch. If you "don't have five minutes," get up five minutes earlier and stop making excuses. In this novena, that's the first attachment we're giving up: excuses. In the prayer portion, we'll also give up our attachments to having to keep busy, to be connected, to do our regular routine. This is five minutes of your day to give God — who, as we mentioned, speaks in "a still small voice" — the space to speak. And to give you space just to listen.

For the workout portion, plan the time for this the night before. If this is the first time in a long time that you've worked out, be sure to do the fitness test from Chapter Two before you begin. But all the workouts for this novena are designed to be done without the need for a gym, in case you haven't gotten around to getting a membership to one yet. Plan out the time frame for each workout the night before, and commit to it. Don't leave the planning for the next day and just say, "I'll see when I can fit it in." I've never met a soul in my life who just "fits in" important things. We fit in errands, deleting our emails, putting gas in the car. Those things can wait for a time of convenience. We don't "fit in" our relationships, whether with God through prayer and Mass or with our family and friends; we don't "fit in" our work; and we don't "fit in" the care of our body. If we don't intentionally set aside time for these things, they won't happen. So, as far as your workout goes, for the following nine days, it is a commitment you make the night before and live out the next day.

DAY 1

PRAYER: Wake up, thank God for three things, then find silence, and sit in that silence for 5 minutes, listening to what God says to you today.

THE HOTEL SPECIAL WORKOUT

This is a 15-minute AMRAP (As Many Reps As Possible). With shorter AMRAPs, we'll go more all-out, but here, go through the following circuit as many times as you can in 15 minutes while keeping your heart rate in the "endurance" range, approximately 180 bpm minus your age. It will definitely spike over that during your Burpees, so wait for it to come down before continuing the workout. So, if you're 35, you'll try to keep your heart rate from about 135–145, but on the Burpees, expect that it will rise up close to your max heart rate of 175–185. Just let it come back down a little before continuing. If you haven't worked out in forever, and even going through the workout once takes longer than 15 minutes, still finish the workout.

- **15 Burpees** (The Burpee utilizes momentum, so ideally I recommend watching a video on it. CrossFitHQ on YouTube has several good ones.)

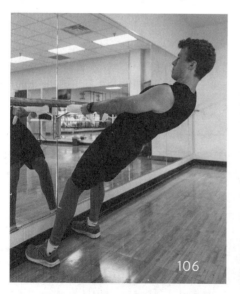 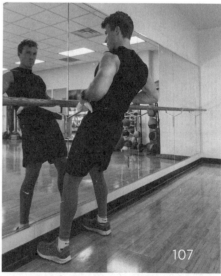

- **10 towel rows** (106, 107) Wrap a towel around a vertical bar (or horizontal if you can't find a vertical one) so that you're holding one end in each hand. Place your feet as close as possible to the bar. Keeping your back slightly arched and shoulders back, pull yourself toward the bar until your hands reach your sides. Hold the contraction and then slowly return to the starting position.

- **5 push-ups** (108, 109) Support your body between your feet and hands. Keep your body in a straight line, and place your hands at a distance apart that will create a 90-degree angle in the middle of the movement between the forearms and the upper arms. Let your body down until your chest touches the floor and then return to the top position. If you can't complete one rep like

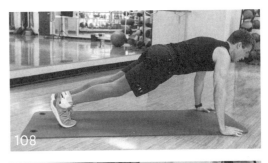
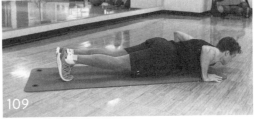

that, support your body in a straight line between your knees and hands instead.

- **25 crunches**

- **Post-workout nutrition**

- **Schedule tomorrow's workout**

DAY 2

PRAYER: Wake up, thank God for three things, find silence, and sit there for 5 minutes... just listening.

GET A LEG UP WORKOUT

We've got another 15-minute AMRAP today. Same idea: even though your heart rate might spike a few times, we're looking to keep it close to your endurance heart rate (180 minus your age) for 15 minutes. If you can get outside for this workout, great, because a little extra space will help.

- **15 air squats** (110, 111) Position your legs shoulder width apart or a little wider, with the toes pointed slightly out. Keeping your head up, core tight, and knees behind your toes at all times, lower your body by bending the knees as you maintain a straight posture and flat back. Continue down until the upper legs are just below parallel to the floor. Push back up to a standing position, again keeping your head up and knees behind the toes.

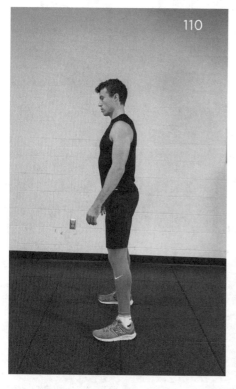
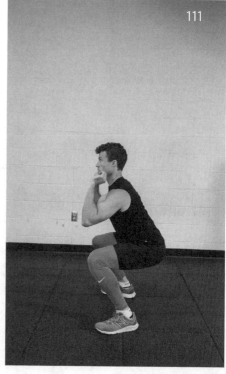

- **5 star jumps** (112, 113) With your feet shoulder width apart and arms close to the body, squat down halfway and explode back up as high as possible. Completely extend your entire body, spreading your legs and arms. As you land, bring your legs and arms back in and absorb your impact through the legs.

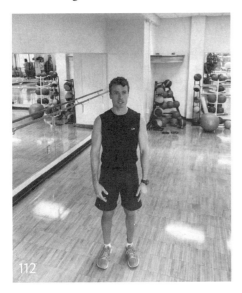
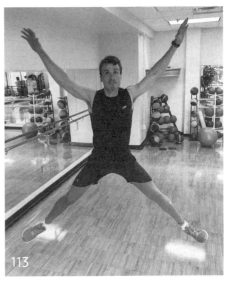

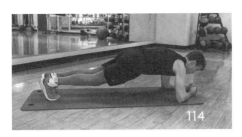
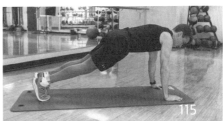

- **30-second plank** (114, 115, 116, 117, 118) Planks can be done with forearms on the ground (standard, 114), or hands on the ground (elevated, 115), which is more challenging. Place toes on the ground and hold yourself

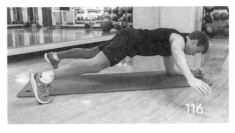

up with your core tight and butt slightly above a straight line between back and legs. You can also do what I like to call "Plank Variations on a Theme," which, as pictured, involves doing 1. a regular plank, 2. one-arm planks on each side (spread legs wider here for balance), 3. side planks each side (stack your feet, keep your body in a straight line, and keep your pelvis up and out), and 4. the "superman" position (lie on your stomach, arch your back, and try to hold your straight arms and legs off the floor).

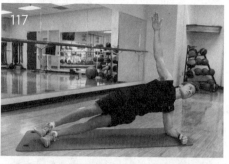

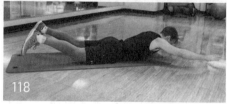

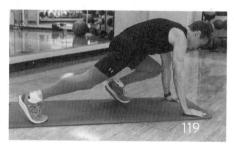

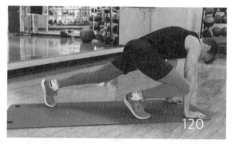

- **20 mountain climbers** (119, 120) From an elevated plank position, place one foot forward. Quickly and explosively switch your feet. Then switch back.

- **10 jumping lunges** (5 each side) Jumping lunges are a movement best learned from a video. I recommend the video "Jumping Lunge Technique" from OFFTHEFIELD on YouTube.

- **Post-workout nutrition**

- **Schedule tomorrow's workout**

DAY 3

PRAYER: Wake up, offer gratitude to God, find silence, sit there and listen for 5 minutes.

ACTIVE RECOVERY

In this novena, we will do two days of workouts, and then one day of active recovery. As you may remember from Chapter Ten on "The Training Trinity," rest serves an invaluable function in training. However, rest doesn't mean being completely sedentary. So, find time to choose activity over total rest: walk, take the stairs, park a block from where you need to go, stretch and do a few jumping jacks at intervals during the day... move at every opportunity.

- **Schedule tomorrow's workout**

DAY 4

PRAYER: Wake up, thank God, eliminate distractions, and listen for God speaking for 5 minutes.

HIT CALISTHENICS PART I

Calisthenics are essentially bodyweight exercises, and we'll incorporate three parts of High Intensity Training into them here: first, every exercise will go to failure, which means you cannot possibly complete another rep. How do you know you can't? Well, because you try to complete a rep for at least 5 seconds before giving up. On that failure rep, you'll also take 10 seconds to do the negative portion of the rep, to be sure you're totally burned out. Second, each rep you do will be very slow: 5 seconds up, 5 seconds down. And third, every set should take at least 1 minute to complete. We'll follow the strength-training portion with a short cardio session.

- **Push-ups, one set to failure**

- **Pull-ups** (or towel rows if pull-ups are not feasible), one set to failure (121,

122) Grab the pull-up bar with palms facing forward, about shoulder width apart. Bring your torso back around 30 degrees or so while sticking your chest out. Pull your torso up until the bar touches your upper chest by drawing the upper arms and shoulder down and back. Return to the bottom of the rep in a controlled manner. Also, the pull-up is a complex movement, but one of the best you can do for your strength and fitness. I recommend watching a video for more detail. My favorite is "The Perfect Pull Up – Do it right!" by CalisthenicMovement on YouTube. I strongly favor strict pull-ups over "kipping" or "butterfly" pull-ups.

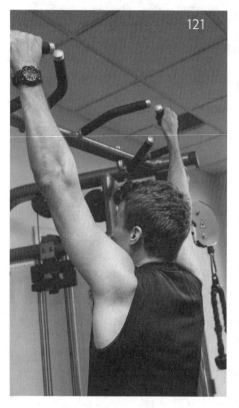 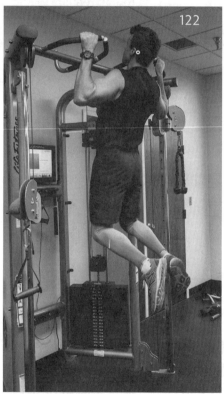

- Crunches, one set to failure

- Jog for at least 12 minutes, staying in endurance heart-rate zone the whole time

- Post-workout nutrition

- Schedule tomorrow's workout

DAY 5

PRAYER: Whether you're growing to love it or growing annoyed by it, prayer is the same today. Wake up, find 5 minutes of silence, and listen.

HIT CALISTHENICS PART II

Same as yesterday, every exercise goes to failure, each rep is 5 seconds up, 5 seconds down, and every set takes at least 1 minute to complete. Since we are heavily working shoulders today, be sure to do 2 minutes of good shoulder warm-up first.

- **Air squats, one set to failure**

- **Handstand push-ups to failure if you have a spotter** (If you don't have a spotter, perform decline push-ups/decline pike push-ups to failure) (123, 124) Position yourself in a handstand either facing toward or away from

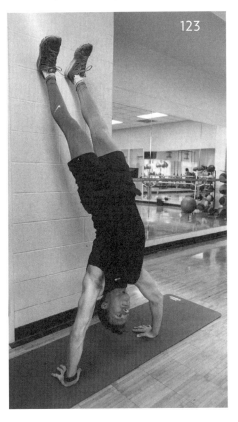
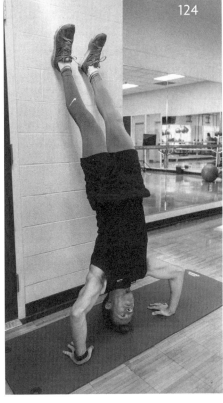

the wall (use a spotter to get into position the first few times your perform the exercise). Your arms and legs should be fully extended and your entire body should be as straight as possible. Keep your head facing forward, rather than down at the ground. Slowly and in control, lower yourself to the ground until your head almost touches the floor. Push yourself back up slowly until your arms are fully extended (but not locked). (125, 126) Decline push-ups are performed the same as a regular push-up, but with feet elevated off the ground. Your hands may be positioned a little further forward than a standard push-up. (127, 128) Pike push-ups are performed similarly to a handstand push-up, with arms extended straight above head and hips angled to place the legs in a triangle shape in relation to the torso. They may be performed on a flat surface or with a sturdy elevated surface to increase intensity.

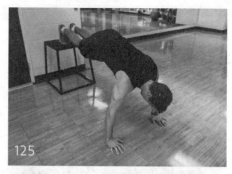

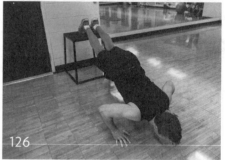

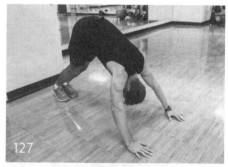

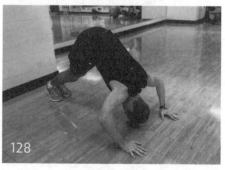

- **Wall sit, one set to failure** (129) Sit with your back flat against a wall and nothing underneath you, legs slightly apart, knees behind your toes and bent at a 90-degree angle.

- **Plank to failure** (advanced can do alternating 15-second one-arm planks to failure)

- **Jog for at least 12 minutes, staying in endurance heart-rate zone the whole time**

- **Post-workout nutrition**

- **Schedule tomorrow's workout**

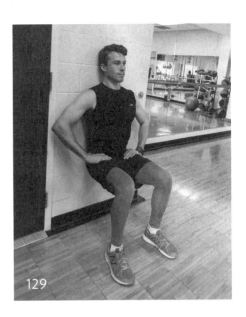

129

DAY 6

PRAYER: Same as before, wake up, thank God, then take 5 minutes of silence to listen to God.

ACTIVE RECOVERY

- **Same as on day three, stay active throughout the day and stretch out any stiffness**

- **Get a gym membership**

- **Seriously. If you haven't done it, go do it.** Find a gym nearby to help minimize your excuses and join. Don't do any of the "Well, I'll get a membership once I've really taken a few decades to get used to exercise," or "I've got to analyze all the possible gyms within a 25-mile radius to make sure I'm getting the best deal," or "I know I'm not going to have time for it anyway" excuse-making. You'll get used to exercise at the gym, you don't need to analyze anything because there's not a major qualitative difference between 95% of gyms, and you'll be making time for exercise, so just go get the membership. It will cost you about $0–$100 to start, and $20–$50 a month. Find a way to do it. If, like my friend I mentioned in Chapter Six, you literally live in a monastery, some other cloistered situation, or are 100 miles from the nearest town, spend that $100 and that $50 a month assembling some strength-training tools for yourself. Order a pull-up bar you can put in a doorway, buy a couple kettlebells of different weights, get an old truck tire and buy a sledgehammer to hit it with and a chain to drag it with. If you want to build a lifetime of fitness, I promise you that you will want better tools to do it with than just "nothing."

- **Schedule tomorrow's workout**

DAY 7

PRAYER: Wake up, thank God for three things, maybe even things you don't normally think of as blessings, then spend 5 minutes of silence listening to God.

KNOCKIN' ON HEAVEN'S DOOR

This is my favorite WOD (workout of the day). It's tough, works your whole body, and is a great means of testing progress. I try to do it at least once every month. You can do it as an AMRAP, or "For Time," and the best part is that you can do it with or without a gym! Now, since you bought a gym membership yesterday (you did, right?), I'm going to give you the gym version of the workout. If you're traveling today (which I'm taking as the only acceptable excuse for not doing this in a gym), I'll include alternate options for gym-specific exercises. Do this for 15 minutes if you're a beginner, 20 minutes if you're intermediate, 30 minutes if you're advanced. Always finish the circuit. So, if you hit 15 minutes on your second time through and still have two exercises left to finish the circuit, do those two exercises, even if it takes you past the 15-minute mark.

- **15% grade run on the treadmill, run 0.15 miles (or find a steep hill and run it 5 times)**
- **15 kettlebell swings** (or grab your carry-on luggage if you're traveling and swing it 15 times) (130, 131, 132) With a flat back but leaning forward,

your core tight and shoulders back, hold a kettlebell between your legs. Thrusting with your hamstrings, drive your hips forward, bringing the kettlebell up using your momentum (not raising slowly with your shoulders). Bring it to shoulder height for a "Russian Swing" or all the way above your head for an "American Swing." Allow the momentum and weight to bring the kettlebell back to the starting position while keeping control of your body. Since this exercise uses momentum, it's great to see a video of it. I recommend CrossFit HQ on YouTube.

•

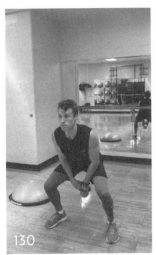 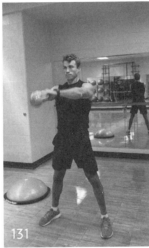 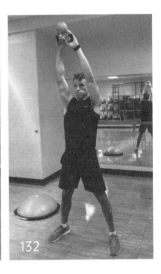

- **15 pull-ups/inverted push-ups** (or towel rows in your hotel room, you jet-setter!) (133, 134) Hang at arms length from a low bar (or TRX handles, as pictured), placing your feet in front of you, with your body as straight as possible. With your back slightly arched and keeping your shoulders back, pull yourself up using your arms and back until your chest touches the bar or handles. Pause briefly and slowly return to your first position.

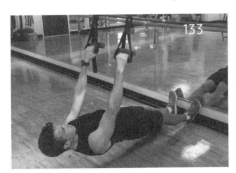 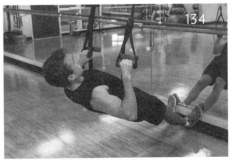

- **15 Burpees**

- **15 goblet squats** (instead of a dumbbell, grab your carry-on, or anything else reasonably heavy) (135, 136) Hold a dumbbell vertically, cradling the top head of it close to your chest with both hands. Position your legs shoulder width apart or a little wider, with toes pointed slightly out. Keeping your head up at all times and your knees behind your toes at all times, lower your body by bending the knees as you maintain a straight posture and flat back. Continue down until the upper legs are just below parallel to the floor. Push back up to a standing position, again keeping your head up and knees behind your toes.

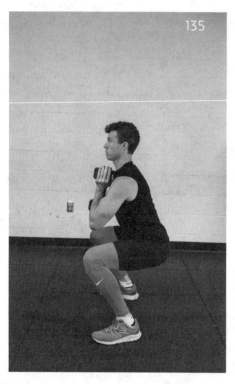
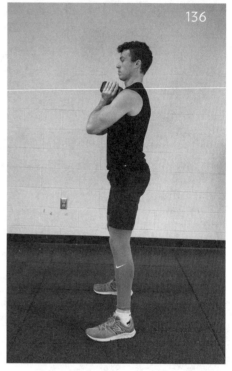

- **Repeat for 15 minutes for beginners, 20 minutes for intermediate, or 30 minutes for advanced**

- **Post-workout nutrition**

- **Schedule tomorrow's workout**

DAY 8

PRAYER: Wake up, give three expressions of thanks, then 5 minutes of silent listening. The *Catechism* says, "The habitual difficulty in prayer is distraction" (2729). So, if you find yourself distracted, that's fine. Just bring your mind back to God and the desire to listen to him.

THE LONG RUN

Okay, I didn't really need to title this workout, because that just describes what this is: a long run. Do a walk/jog/run (depending on your level of fitness) for 45–90 minutes (depending on your level of fitness). Keep your heart rate in the endurance zone. We're not concerned about distance or speed, just about time and heart rate. I really prefer trail running, but you can run on the road if necessary, or on an elliptical or treadmill. Just please don't run on a sidewalk. Your bones and joints will thank you. Trails keep me interested, relaxed, and engaged, and they provide enough variation that you can keep your heart rate in the right zone, whether that means jogging, running, or walking/hiking. I find interest and relaxation harder to sustain during 90 minutes on a treadmill. But work with what you have access to; put in the time and keep your heart rate in the right zone.

- Post-workout nutrition

- Schedule tomorrow's workout

DAY 9

PRAYER: I hope that expressing gratitude and taking 5 minutes of silent prayer each morning have become something you love and helps start your day on the right foot. If not, well, no one's forcing you to do them past this novena, so today's your last day! Either way, today, wake up, thank God and spend 5 minutes in silence, listening to him.

ACTIVE RECOVERY

Today, after yesterday's long cardio session, be sure you're doing what you need to do to get proper nutrition, hydration, etc., to recover from your workout. Also keep stretching and keep moving so you don't get stiff. If it was particularly taxing, you might even consider taking an Epsom soak for your legs, or an ice bath, to help your legs bounce back more quickly.

- **Schedule tomorrow's workout**

- **Wait, isn't this novena done? Yes, it is... but your life isn't.** I'd encourage you to look at the next longer session of workouts, 21 Days to Build a Habit, as a good continuation! I hope the past nine days have given you more motivation and have gotten you excited to dive in and do more!

21 DAYS TO BUILD A HABIT

You may have heard the adage that it takes 21 days to build a new habit — but where did that come from? Well, in the 1950s, a plastic surgeon named Dr. Maxwell Maltz saw that it took most of his patients about three weeks to get used to their new appearance, and in 1960 he wrote a book called *Psycho-Cybernetics*, where he theorized that we could more broadly say that it takes at minimum 21 days to change our mental images, integral to building new habits.

That book sold 30 million or so copies, so the concept of building a habit in 21 days took hold, even though Dr. Maltz himself used that as a *minimum*. More research has shown that habits often vary widely in how long they take to build (between two to eight months on average) and how persistent they are. However, 21 days still serves as a great minimum starting point.

When it comes to prayer, perseverance really is the key. As we noted in the last chapter, the Catechism says "The habitual difficulty in prayer is distraction." When we experience this, our response needs to be one of reorienting ourselves to God. Whether that means just bringing our focus back, or taking time in silence, or going to confession, we need to look for the opportunity to come back to God as often as we stray.

In this workout plan, we're working on building a habit, which incidentally leads us to again mention the *Catechism's* definition of virtue: "A virtue is an habitual and firm disposition to do the good. It allows the person not only to perform good acts, but to give the best of himself" (1803). So we possess a virtue when we habitually choose the good of that virtue (courage in the face of fear, temperance when confronted with excess, kindness instead of anger, and so on.

So for this session we'll be focusing on practicing virtuous acts every day. Obviously, we want to embody all the virtues every day, but again we're trying to build a habit of taking measurable action daily, so we'll focus on one main virtue each day. Sometimes when one of the cardinal virtues (courage, justice, temperance, prudence) or theological virtues (faith, hope, charity) pairs up nicely with one of the seven "heavenly" virtues (the list of virtues directly opposed to the seven deadly sins), I'll include that as well, so, you know, keep an eye out.

In the physical workouts, you'll notice we start at Day 10. Why is that? Because you've done the previous nine workouts, right? If you haven't, start with those and come back here afterward. Now that we've laid a base of fitness, we'll take the rest of these 21 days to begin rotating the kind of training we're doing, so that we're working on all the components of fitness longer term. Don't worry, we'll have rest days built in, so you'll be able to work that fitness component as well!

DAY 10

PRAYER: I still encourage gratitude and 5 minutes of silence, but now each day we'll also be focusing on one or more of the virtues. Today's virtues are charity and chastity.

Charity is "the theological virtue by which we love God above all things for his own sake, and our neighbor as ourselves for the love of God" (CCC 1822). Closely allied to that is chastity. Chastity doesn't just mean "not having sex" or "not lusting"; it's much bigger than that. "Chastity means the successful integration of sexuality within the person and thus the inner unity of man in his bodily and spiritual being" (CCC 2337). Chastity is our love lived out fully. A spiritual director of mine told me that chastity is a true expression of our creative function, in the fullest sense. When we yield to temptation to lust, we're avoiding sharing in the creation of God.

Today then, if you're tempted to "unchastity," reorient yourself. Often the best way to do that is what I'm going to suggest for your virtuous act today: create. Make of yourself a gracious gift of self. Make dinner for someone. Read 1 Corinthians 13, or a paragraph of *Deus Caritas Est* by Pope Benedict XVI, or *Love and Responsibility* by Pope Saint John Paul II; then spend 5 minutes writing a meditation on what you read. Write a love letter to your husband or wife. Be creative in an expression of pure, life-giving love to someone. You've got a lot of options. Pick one and do it!

"CHESTITY"

Please forgive the atrocious pun. This week we're focusing on strength and incorporating the concept of "splits." Rather than working out your whole body, you split it up to focus on different body parts on different days. Today, you guessed it, we'll be working on chest (and also shoulders and triceps). Beginner, intermediate, and advanced will all do the same amount of sets, just with different weight.

- Warm up your shoulders, which are a joint particularly prone to injury, by doing arms circles and some raises and rotations with very light weight

- 10–15 push-ups or knee push-ups (keep it easy) just as a warm up for chest. Or if that's too challenging, pick a super-light weight and do bench presses with that for 10–15.

- **Clean and press, 3 sets.** Pick a weight you could do 8–10 reps with, but just do 5 reps. Rest 2 minutes, repeat 2 more times, for a total of 3 sets. Clean and press is a movement that utilizes momentum, and the best way to learn the form is through watching a video. I recommend the ones either from Bodybuilding.com or CrossFit HQ on YouTube.

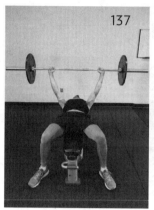 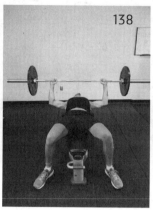 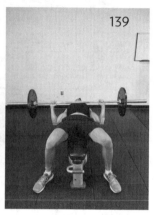

- **Bench press, 4 sets.** Frequently with strength training, we'll do percentages of our ORM or One-Rep Max. This term refers to the most weight with which you could successfully complete 1 rep. We'll almost never actually lift that weight, but we'll lift percentages of it. Try to gauge what that would be (err on the side of lighter rather than heavier — that is, if you think it's somewhere between 100 and 150, go with 100. If that's too easy, go heavier next time). Then do the following: 1 set at 60% ORM for 5 reps (notated as 1x60%x5), 1x65%x5, 2x75%x5 (2 sets at 75% for 5 reps). Rest for 2.5 minutes following each set. (137, 138, 139) Lie back on a flat bench. Using a grip that creates a 90-degree angle in the middle of the movement between the forearms and the upper arms, lift the bar from the rack and hold it straight over your chest with your arms locked and shoulders back. Bring the bar down slowly until the bar touches your midchest, then push the bar back to the starting position, focusing on pushing the bar using your chest muscles.

- **Incline dumbbell bench press, 1 set.** Here we are going to failure, so find someone to spot you. For safety, we're going to keep it in a slightly higher rep range. You'll do 50% of your ORM for 8–12 reps. Each rep will be done slowly, 2 seconds up, 4 seconds down. (140, 141, 142, 143) Using an incline bench or an adjustable bench set at 30–45 degrees, hold two dumbbells and perform the same pressing motion as in regular bench

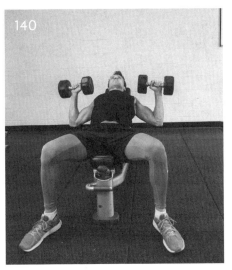
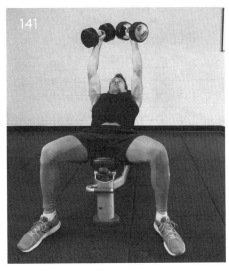
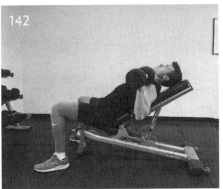
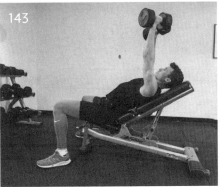

press. There are two minor differences. First, at the top of the rep, to get full use of the range of motion allowed by dumbbells, bring the dumbbells into an A-shape rather than just straight across. Second, at the bottom of the rep, because you're on an incline, the dumbbells should be just higher than your midchest.

- **Super-slow push-ups, 1 set.** Rest 30 seconds after completing your dumbbell bench press, then do push-ups until failure, 5 seconds up, 5 seconds down. You may only be able to do 1 or 2, or you might get up to 5 or 6, but since you went to failure on your last exercise, it shouldn't be much more than that before you really can't complete another rep.

- **Dumbbell shoulder press, 4 sets.** Here, just pick a manageable weight and do 4 sets of 10 reps apiece with a 1-minute rest following each set. It should be very challenging by the end of the fourth set. (144, 145) Stand with your feet shoulder width apart and a dumbbell in each hand at head height, the elbows out just under 90 degrees. While remaining standing straight up, facing forward, extend your arms to raise the weights together directly above your head.

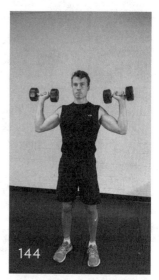

144

- **Superset of tricep dips/push-downs, 3 sets.** Two superset exercises, we do them back-to-back without rest in between. Do 10 reps of dips, then switch immediately to 12 reps of push-downs, then rest 1 minute. Do that all again. And again. "Superset:" is how you'll see it noted from now on.

- **Tricep dips 3x10** (146, 147) Place a bench or box behind your back and perpendicular to your body, and a second box or bench (ideally of equal height) under your feet, legs fully extended and perpendicular to your torso. Grip the bench with both hands, about shoulder width apart. Slowly lower your body by bending at the elbows until there is an angle slightly smaller than 90 degrees between the upper arm and the forearm, keeping the elbows close to your body throughout the movement. Push your body up using your triceps to return to your starting position.

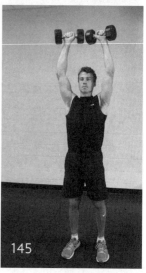

145

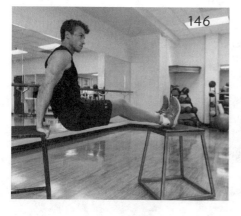

146

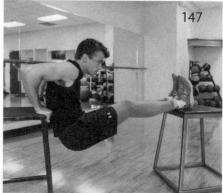

147

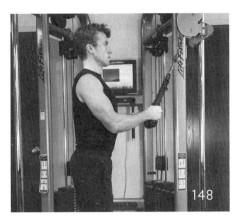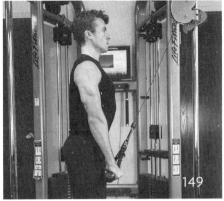

- **Rope push-downs, 3x12** (148, 149) Connect a rope attachment to a high pulley and hold with your palms facing each other. Keeping your back flat, with a slight lean forward, and your elbows close to your body, use your triceps to push the rope down until your hands are basically at your sides. Then return the rope slowly up to the starting point.

- **Rest 1 minute 3 times**

- **Optional: Quad-set of lateral raise, front raise, rear raise, and press, 4 sets.** A quad-set, as you might guess, is 4 exercises back-to-back without rest (and yes, 3 is a tri-set). Do 8 reps of all of these in a row. (You may need to do lighter weights for the lateral and front raise than you used for the rear raise and presses.) Rest 1 minute. Do it all 4 times.

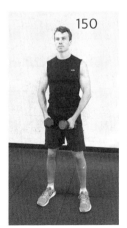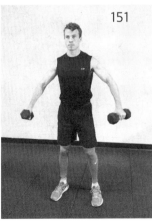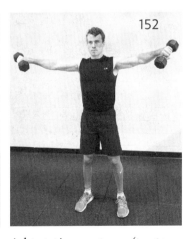

- **Lateral raise, 4x8** (150, 151, 152) With an upright stationary torso (try to avoid swinging), lift dumbbells from your side with a slight bend on the elbow and the hands slightly tilted forward as if pouring water from a pitcher. Continue to go up until your arms are parallel to the floor. Pause briefly and return slowly to the bottom of the rep.

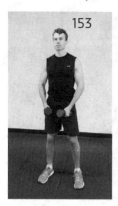 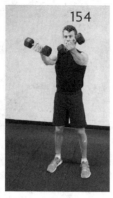 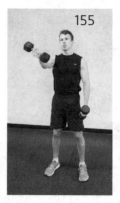 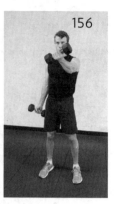

- **Front raise, 4x8** (153, 154, 155, 156) With an upright stationary torso (try to avoid swinging), lift dumbbells from your side with a slight bend on the elbow and turn the palms up through the rep. Continue to go up until your arms are parallel to the floor. Pause briefly and return slowly to the bottom of the rep. This can be done together or by alternating arms.

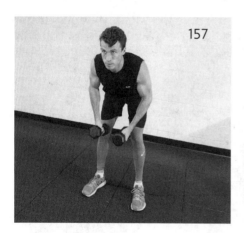 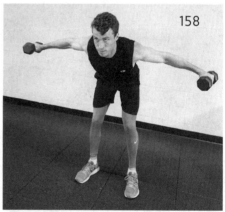

- **Rear raise, 4x8** (157, 158) Bending at the hip with a straight back at a 30-degree angle from the floor, lift dumbbells from your side with a slight bend on the elbow and the hands slightly tilted forward as if pouring water from a pitcher. Continue to go up until your arms are parallel to the floor. Pause briefly and return slowly to the bottom of the rep.

- Dumbbell shoulder press, 4x8

- Rest 1 minute

- **Stretch your shoulders, chest, and triceps ballistically to cool down, then do a couple of static stretches, then a little more ballistic stretching.** You can also opt to do 15–20 minutes of low intensity cardio (endurance level heart rate) here.

- Schedule tomorrow's workout

DAY 11

PRAYER: Gratitude and 5 minutes of silence. Fortitude "is the moral virtue that ensures firmness in difficulties and constancy in the pursuit of the good. It strengthens the resolve to resist temptations and to overcome obstacles in the moral life" (CCC 1808). What do you find difficult, not in the short run, but in the long haul? Is it because you tend to take on too much at once? Or because you are easily bored and are always looking for something new? Or just worn down? Commit to consistency in something small today, like making your bed, or shutting off the lights.

"LEG-ENDARY"

Oh gosh, the puns get worse. This one doesn't even have anything to do with the virtue! Luckily, the workout does have something to do with the virtue. Legs are *way* stronger than most people give them credit for. Your top three largest and strongest muscle groups are all in your legs: your glutes, your hamstrings, and your quadriceps. Whenever my brain thinks I can't do any more leg work, I know that always means I've got at least 2 more reps in me. With that in mind, exercise your fortitude by pushing yourself to get the reps, the range of motion, and the sets you fear in today's workout. Your legs can take it, get your mind on board!

- **Spend 5 minutes on the treadmill to warm up.** Walk uphill, go sideways and backward if you feel comfortable doing it (at very low speeds)!

- **Air squats to warm up.** Stretch your legs throughout the workout.

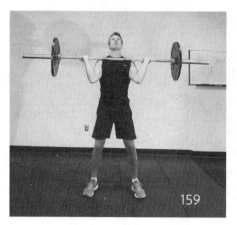

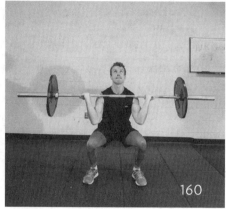

- **Front squats, 4 sets. 60% ORMx5, 65%x5, 75%x5, 75%x5.** Rest 2.5 minutes after each set. (159, 160) Put the barbell into a "rack position," where you rest the bar on your shoulder muscles (deltoids), keeping the elbows high and the upper arm slightly above parallel to the floor. Position your legs shoulder width apart with toes pointed forward or slightly out. Keeping your head up, core tight, and knees behind your toes at all times, lower your body by bending the knees as you maintain a straight posture and flat back. Continue down until the upper legs are just below parallel to the floor. Push back up to a standing position, again keeping your head up and knees behind the toes.

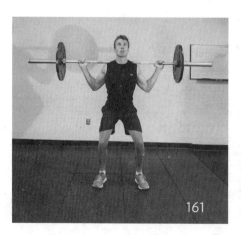

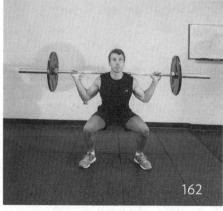

- **Squats, 4 sets. 40–50% ORM for 8–12 reps.** As on chest day, each rep should be done slowly: 2 seconds up, 4 seconds down. One minute rest between sets. (161, 162) With a barbell resting across your upper back and shoulders (just below your neck), position your legs shoulder width apart or a little wider, with toes pointed slightly out. Keeping your head up, core tight, and knees behind your toes at all times, lower your body by bending the knees as you maintain a straight posture and flat back. Continue down until the upper legs are just below parallel to the floor. Push back up to a standing position, again keeping your head up and knees behind the toes.

SUPERSET:

- **Single leg press, 4x8–12**

- **Leg press calf raise, 4x30.** Instead of an actual rest period after single leg press, just do 30 quick reps of calf raise on the leg press, 10 reps regular, 10 reps toes in, and 10 reps toes out. Then back to single leg press! (163, 164) Push a leg press platform until your legs are almost straight (just don't lock your knees). Position your feet about shoulder width, with the balls of your feet just above the edge of the platform, and your heels hanging beneath. Press on the platform by pushing the balls of your feet down and raising your heels, flexing your calf. Keep your knees stationary (but not locked) at all times. Hold the contracted position for a second before returning to the bottom of the rep. You may adjust your toe position between toes pointing forward, pointing out, and pointing in.

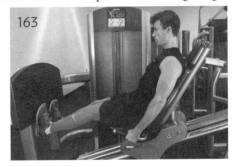
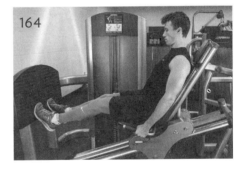

TRI-SET:

- **Seated calf raise, 4x30** (again, each set is 10 reps regular, 10 toes in, 10 toes out)

- **Bosu crunches, 4x10–40** (There's a big rep range here, because I want you to go almost to failure. That may be 10 reps for some people, 40 or more for others. Do your best.) (165, 166, 167) Lie with your mid to low back on a Bosu. Elevate and squeeze your glutes, and keep your knees out and strong. Crunch straight up, bringing your torso toward the ceiling (not curling into your legs). Return slowly to the bottom of the rep, but keep your abs tight the whole time, even while carefully stretching your back over the ball. Don't use your hands to pull, don't relax your abs even at the bottom of the rep.

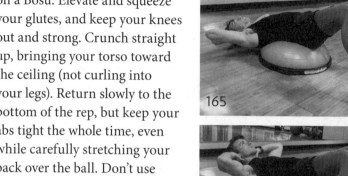

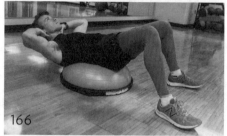

- **Plank, 1 minute.** If a plank for one minute is too hard, do it from your knees. If it's too easy, do a one-arm plank for 30 seconds each side.

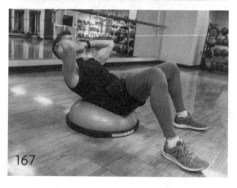

- **Cool down/stretch!** Walk on the treadmill for 2 minutes, take 5 minutes to do some ballistic and static stretching. You can also optionally do 15–20 minutes of low intensity cardio (endurance level heart rate) here.

- **Schedule tomorrow's workout**

DAY 12

PRAYER: Gratitude and 5 minutes of silence. Today's virtue is justice. "Justice is the moral virtue that consists in the constant and firm will to give their due to God and neighbor" (CCC 1807). What will you be doing today? Well, usually, our fallen nature tends to leave us erring on the side of thinking that people "deserve" less than they do, and acting in accordance with that. So, today, treat everyone with whom you come in contact a little better than you normally would. Make an extra effort. Give your kids more attention, praise an employee or coworker you overlook, give your mom or dad a call just to talk. Find a way to show love and respect, and do it.

BACK BEHIND BARS

Starting tomorrow, I'm not even going to comment on the names of these workouts, but today I'll just say, man, this one may be my worst attempt at keeping the workout relevant to the virtue.

- **Warm up with some jumping jacks, rowing machine, maybe a couple of bodyweight pull-ups.** Get your arms and your back warm. And it's always a good idea to warm your shoulders up a little more.

- **Pull-ups/weighted pull-ups.** If you can get more than 8 pull-ups in a row, do weighted pull-ups. Rest 2.5 minutes after each set.

- **Barbell row:** (171, 168, 169, 170) Holding a barbell with an overhand grip, bend your knees slightly and bring your torso forward, by bending at the waist, while keeping the back straight until it is between 45 degrees and almost parallel to the floor. Keeping your head up, shoulders back, and

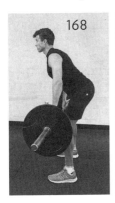
168
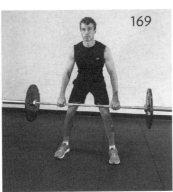
169
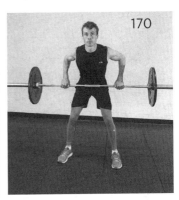
170

elbows close to the body, lift the barbell to you. Briefly pause and then slowly lower the barbell back to the starting position.

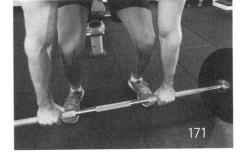
171

- **Incline dumbbell row, 4 sets.**
  50% ORM for 8–12 reps.
  Controlled reps: 2 seconds up,

4 seconds down. One minute rest between sets. (172, 173) Lean into an incline bench, with a dumbbell in each hand, shoulders back. Row the dumbbells to your side, pause slightly at the top, and then return to the starting position.

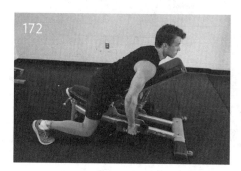
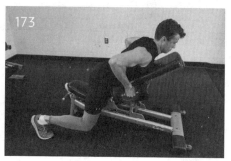

- **Inverted push-ups, 4 sets, 8–12 reps.** Position your feet where you need to in order to complete the set. One minute rest between sets.

TRI-SET FOR BICEPS:

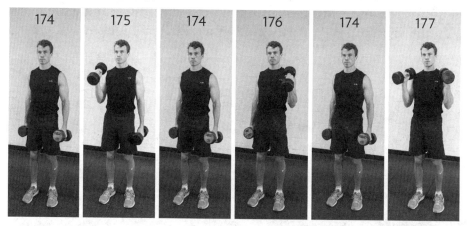

- **Hammer curl 4x8** (174, 175, 174 again, 176, 174 again, 177) Stand with your torso upright and a dumbbell in each hand with palms facing your torso. While holding the upper arm stationary, curl one dumbbell straight up, using the bicep. Continue the movement until your bicep is fully contracted and the dumbbell is at shoulder level. Hold the contracted position for a second as you squeeze the bicep, then return slowly to the bottom of the rep. Repeat on the other side. That is one rep. You can also perform this exercise both arms at once rather than alternating.

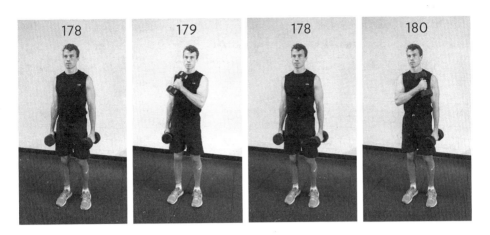

- **Cross body curl 4x8** (178, 179, 178 again, 180) Stand with your torso upright and a dumbbell in each hand with palms facing your torso. While holding the upper arm stationary, curl one dumbbell up and across the body to the opposite shoulder, using the bicep. Continue the movement until your bicep is fully contracted and the dumbbell is at shoulder level. Hold the contracted position for a second as you squeeze the bicep, then return slowly to the bottom of the rep. Repeat on the other side. That is one rep.

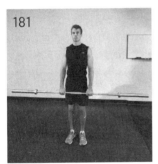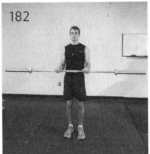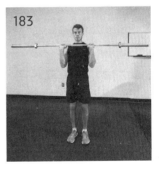

- **Reverse barbell curl 4x8** (181, 182, 183) Stand up with your torso upright, holding a barbell at shoulder width with the elbows close to the torso. The palm of your hands should be facing down. Keeping the upper arms stationary and moving only the forearms, curl the weights while contracting the biceps. Continue the movement until your biceps are fully contracted and the bar is at your shoulder level. Hold the contracted position for a second, then slowly begin to bring the bar back to the bottom of the rep.

- **Stretch your back and biceps, ballistically to cool down, then a couple of static stretches, then a little more ballistic stretching.** You can also optionally do 15–20 minutes of low intensity cardio (endurance level heart rate) here.

- **Schedule tomorrow's workout**

DAY 13

PRAYER: Gratitude and 5 minutes of silence. Today's virtue is temperance. Temperance moderates our desire for pleasure so we're not controlled by our urges. Today, pick something you know you want and give it up. Keep it simple. If you like or love meat (as I do), abstain from meat for the day. Give up sweets if that's your poison, or Facebook or Instagram for the day. Again, we're picking something that provides pleasure (which is a good), and sacrificing it. Picking a sin to give up doesn't count. We'll also be incorporating a rest day today to be sure we exercise restraint in our workout, too.

ACTIVE RECOVERY

Be sure you're doing what you need to do to get proper nutrition, hydration, etc., to properly recover from your workouts. Also keep stretching and keep moving, so you don't get stiff. Find time to choose activity over total rest: walk, take the stairs, park a block from where you need to go, stretch and do a few jumping jacks at intervals during the day. Just move at every opportunity.

- **Schedule tomorrow's workout**

DAY 14

PRAYER: Gratitude and 5 minutes of silence. Faith is "the theological virtue by which we believe in God and believe all that he has said and revealed to us, and that Holy Church proposes for our belief, because he is truth itself" (CCC 1814). For prayer today, find a way to make the truth God has revealed through the Church your own. To me, the simplest way to do that is to go pray in front of the Blessed Sacrament, even just for a few minutes. It doesn't have to be where the Blessed Sacrament is exposed in Eucharistic Adoration; just find an open church, and if the little red candle is lit, Jesus is there in the tabernacle. Go sit with him.

DROP 'TIL YOU STOP

Today we're upping the volume of reps we're doing, a great way to work strength a little differently. Start by warming up your shoulders and core, then warm up the rest of your body as well, I like doing 3 tiny sets of Burpees (maybe 3–5 each) for that.

- **Incline dumbbell bench 4x5+5.** What does that notation mean? It means you'll do 5 reps at a challenging weight, then drop the amount of weight 10% and go again immediately. You'll rest 2.5 minutes, then repeat the set, for a total of 4 sets.

- **Incline dumbbell row 4x5+5.** You guessed it, same thing here: do the first 5 reps, drop the weight 10%, go again, rest 2.5 minutes.

SUPERSET FOR CHEST AND BACK 1X10+10+10+10:

- **Cable crossover, high to low.** (184, 185) Put the cable pulleys in a high position, step slightly forward of the pulleys, with a slight bend in your waist and in your elbows. Rotating from your shoulder, bring your arms in front of you in a wide

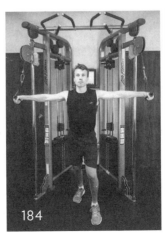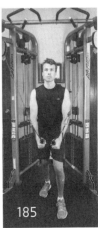

arc until your hands are both low and in front of you. Squeeze and then slowly return your arms to their starting position. Do all 4 drops right in a row then move on.

- **Cable row.** (186, 187) Either sit on the ground or get into an elevated squat position. Using almost any cable attachment (my favorites are the rope, as pictured, or the v-bar) and keeping your back slightly arched and shoulders back, pull the

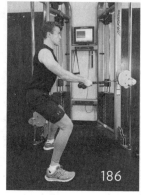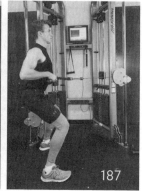

handle back toward you until it touches or almost touches your stomach. Hold the contraction and then slowly return the weight to the starting position. Do all 4 drops in a row.

- **Rest 2.5 minutes**

SUPERSET FOR ARMS 1X10+10+10+10:
- **Tricep push-downs**

- **Cable curl.** (188, 189, 190, 191, 190 again, 192) Stand upright while holding a cable curl bar that is attached to a low pulley (or two cable handles on two low pulleys). Grab the cable bar at shoulder width and keep the elbows close to the torso, with the palms of your hands facing up. While holding the upper arms stationary (move only the forearms), contract the biceps to curl the weights.

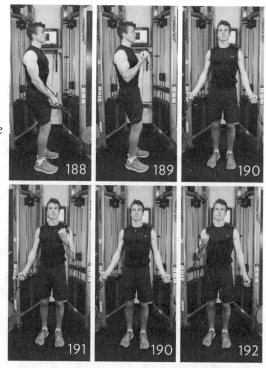

Continue the movement until your biceps are fully contracted and the bar is at shoulder level. Squeeze the contracted position for a second and then return to your first position. This exercise can be done with alternating curls if two independent handles are used.

- **Stretch.** Some ballistic, some static. You can also optionally do 15–20 minutes of low intensity cardio (endurance level heart rate) here.

- **Schedule tomorrow's workout**

DAY 15

PRAYER: Gratitude and 5 minutes of silence. Hope is "the theological virtue by which we desire the kingdom of heaven and eternal life as our happiness, placing our trust in Christ's promises and relying not on our own strength, but on the help of the grace of the Holy Spirit" (CCC 1817). The *Catechism* goes on to say that Christian hope unfolds in the beatitudes. So, to get practical with hope, pick a beatitude and live that out today. Remember that you're the one called to be poor in spirit, or mourning, or meek, etc. You're not supposed to go find someone else who is. So, mourn if you have the occasion to, be merciful, make peace, be pure, hunger for righteousness! For your reference, here is Matthew's account of the beatitudes:

> Blessed are the poor in spirit, for theirs is the kingdom of heaven.
> Blessed are those who mourn, for they shall be comforted.
> Blessed are the meek, for they shall inherit the earth.
> Blessed are those who hunger and thirst for righteousness, for
> they shall be satisfied.
> Blessed are the merciful, for they shall obtain mercy.
> Blessed are the pure in heart, for they shall see God.
> Blessed are the peacemakers, for they shall be called sons of God.
> Blessed are those who are persecuted for righteousness' sake, for
> theirs is the kingdom of heaven.
> Blessed are you when men revile you and persecute you and utter
> all kinds of evil against you falsely on my account. Rejoice
> and be glad, for your reward is great in heaven, for so men
> persecuted the prophets who were before you. (5:3–12)

POSTERIOR CHAIN GANG

- **Warm up with Bosu crunches and a quick plank "variations on a theme" (nothing too strenuous).** Also do hip thrusters for glute activation. Yes, they look awkward. Yes, they'll prevent injury.

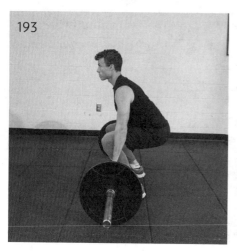

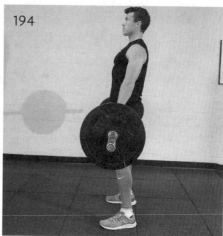

- **Dead lifts, 4 sets.** 60% ORMx5, 65%x5, 75%x5, 75%x5. Rest 2.5 minutes after each set. (195, 193, 194) Place your feet hip width apart, with your knees behind your toes and your grip (one hand overhand, the other underhand) just outside your

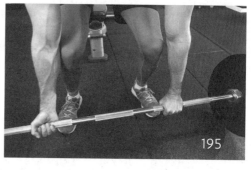

legs. Keeping your back flat and your shoulders back and down, stand up, moving your hips and knees together to the bar from the ground to an upper-thigh, locked position. Keep the bar close to or in contact with your legs at all times

- **Romanian dead lift, 4 sets, 50% ORM for 8–12 reps.** Controlled reps: 2 seconds up, 4 seconds down. One minute rest between sets. (196, 197) Hold a bar at hip level with an overhand grip, keeping your shoulders back, your back slightly arched, and your knees slightly bent. Lower the bar by moving your butt back as far as you can, while keeping the bar close to your body, your head looking forward, and your shoulders back. Lower the bar until just below your knees, then return to the starting position by driving the hips forward to stand up.

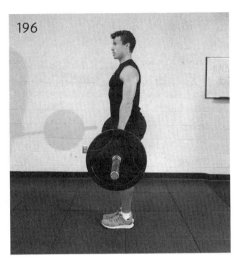
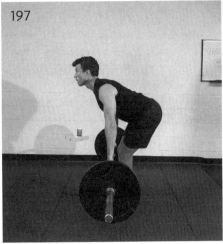

- **Kettlebell (or dumbbell, if you must) swings, 4 sets, 8–12 reps.** One minute rest between sets.

SUPERSET:
- **Bosu crunches, 2 sets to failure**

- **Plank "variations on a theme," 2 sets**

- **Stretch.** Some ballistic, some static. You can also optionally do 15–20 minutes of low intensity cardio (endurance level heart rate) here.

- **Schedule tomorrow's workout**

DAY 16

PRAYER: Gratitude and 5 minutes of silence. Today's virtue is prudence, which is "the virtue that disposes practical reason to discern our true good in every circumstance and to choose the right means of achieving it…. Prudence is 'right reason in action,' writes Saint Thomas Aquinas, following Aristotle…. It guides the other virtues by setting rule and measure" (CCC 1806). Today provides us an opportunity to live out all the other virtues in small ways. At every opportunity today, try to pick the best good, not just any good. When you're working, work without distraction. When you're with your family or friends, give them your full attention, and do the same in your prayer today.

And today is a day of rest... so appreciate that. Eat well, drink water, etc. Bring mindfulness to everything you do. If you notice yourself falling short, don't beat yourself up. Just gently bring your mind and heart back to what you're doing.

ACTIVE RECOVERY

- **Get proper nutrition, hydration, etc., to properly recover from your workouts.** Also keep stretching and keep moving. Walk, take the stairs, move.

- **Schedule tomorrow's workout**

DAY 17

PRAYER: Gratitude and 5 minutes of silence. We're back on charity today. As before, find ways to love, to be creative, and exercise chastity. Today, though, be creative with whom you show love. This time, consider choosing someone you don't find easy to love.

THE POWER OF LOVE

We're jumping into my favorite kind of workouts: powerlifting/Olympic lifting plus a WOD! Get it? I love *power*lifting... never mind, I promised I wouldn't dwell on the names.

- **Warm up legs, shoulders, core**

- **Clean and press 3x5.** Rest 2 minutes between sets.

- **Front squat 3x5.** Rest 2 minutes between sets

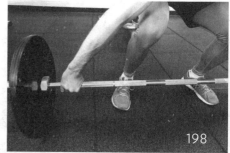

- **Snatch pull: 3x5** (198) This is exactly like a dead lift, except with hands spread as far apart on the barbell as you can get them and still hold on safely.

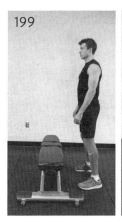 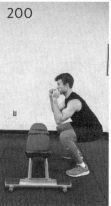 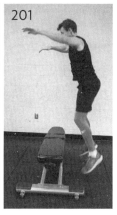 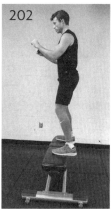

- **EMOM**, **10 mins:**
    - On the even minutes (0, 2, 4, 6, 8), do 10 pull-ups, or substitute inverted push-ups or towel rows if pull-ups aren't feasible.
    - On the odd minutes (1, 3, 5, 7, 9), do 10 squat jumps. If that's too easy, hold a medicine ball or kettlebell to add weight. If it's too challenging for now, do step-ups. (199, 200, 201, 202) Keeping your head up and your back straight, position your feet shoulder width apart. With your back straight and chest up, squat down until your upper thighs are parallel, or lower, to the floor. Now jump straight up in the air as high as possible, using the thighs like springs. You can simply jump in place, or if you feel safe doing it, onto a box or bench. When you touch the floor again, immediately squat down and jump again. For step-ups, use a bench, but instead of jumping up onto it, simply step up, one foot at a time, alternating the first foot each rep.

- **Stretch.** Wow! Isn't this great? A tough workout and it only took a half-hour! Amazing! Love it!

- **Schedule tomorrow's workout**

DAY 18

PRAYER: Gratitude and 5 minutes of silence. We're focusing on faith again today, so sit with the Eucharist, or go to Mass, or maybe just learn something more about a Church teaching you want to understand but don't, or one you have a hard time accepting.

LEG DAY EVERY DAY

Remember how I said your legs are way stronger than you think they are? With these bigger lifts, your legs will generally get worked at least somewhat each day. Today they'll get worked a lot.

- **Warm up by walking forward, sideways, and backward, and stretching a little.** Always warm up shoulders and core as well!

- **Squat cleans, 4x4.** Rest 2 minutes between sets.

- **Squats, 3x4.** Rest 2 minutes between sets.

- **Romanian dead lifts, 2x4.** Rest 2 minutes between sets.

- **AMRAP for 10 minutes: Do all four exercises in a row, then immediately start over.** Do that as many times as possible in 10 minutes. You can rest if you need to, but again, your goal is to get as many times through as possible!

- **20 mountain climbers**

- **5 Burpees**

- **15 air squats**

- **30-second plank**

- **Stretch and cool down**

- **Schedule tomorrow's workout**

DAY 19

PRAYER: Gratitude and 5 minutes of silence. It's hope again today! That means it's time to dive into the beatitudes once more, so get on it!

POWER BACK AND CHEST

- **Pause bench 3x5.** If there aren't stops on your bench press or power rack, get on a chest-press machine, position the handles so that your elbows are at 90 degrees at the bottom of the rep. Either way, at the bottom of your rep, set the weight down completely, then push it back up from a dead stop. Rest 2 minutes between sets.

- **Pause barbell row 3x5.** Again, either do this with the safety stops set on a power rack, or find somewhere slightly elevated but stable where you can set your barbell so that at the bottom of the rep your arms are extended. Then between every rep, you'll set it down just long enough to pick it up from a dead stop. Rest 2 minutes between sets.

SUPERSET:

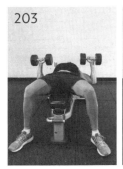 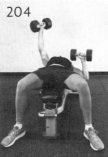 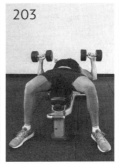 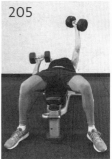

- **Alternating dumbbell bench, 2x8–10** (203, 204, 203 again, 205) Perform the movement the same way you would with a bench press, but with dumbbells. Do one full rep with one arm, then do one full rep with the other arm, using the bottom of the rep as your starting position.

- **Alternating incline dumbbell row, 2x8–10**

- **Rest one minute**

- **For time: Complete the following in any order, split up the sets if you need to, just finish as fast as you can safely!**

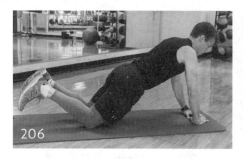 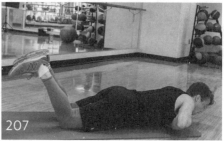

- **30 narrow push-ups (go to your knees if you need to)** (206, 207) Same as regular push-up, but move your hand to narrower position, even touching if you're able. At the bottom of the rep, your hands should touch the center of your chest (giving this push-up variation its other name "heart to heart."

- **25 pull-ups** (assisted or inverted push-ups, if you need to)

- **15 Burpees**

- **50 Bosu crunches**

- **Stretch and cool down**

- **Plan tomorrow's workout**

DAY 20

PRAYER: Today we focus on temperance again… rest, relax, focus on exercising moderation.

ACTIVE RECOVERY

- Plan tomorrow's workout

- Well, you actually get to do active recovery tomorrow as well, but I promise you'll want it!

DAY 21

PRAYER: Gratitude and 5 minutes of silence. It may seem soon, but today is the last day of our 21-day session. We focus on prudence again. Today, think about a choice or decision you need to make. Ask God to guide you to make the choice prudently. Be present, connected, and focused.

ACTIVE RECOVERY

- You know what this looks like at this point! Be active, but recover from three really challenging workouts in a row.

- Plan tomorrow's workout

Yep! Guess what! There are 40- and 90-day plans coming up! Get excited!

40 DAYS IN THE DESERT

Everyone experiences temptation. There may be time in our lives when we are tempted to major sins: adultery, murder, major theft, blasphemy. There will be many more times when we are tempted to the easier versions of those sins: lust in the heart, hatred or wrath, stealing or cheating, cursing and being careless with the name of God. But even more often than that, we experience the smaller temptations and struggles that the world bombards us with daily. We are constantly tempted in a hundred ways to take what we perceive as "the easy way," rather than choosing the good way.

In Matthew 4:1, the Evangelist says that after his baptism by John, "Jesus was led up by the Spirit into the wilderness to be tempted by the devil." Jesus goes into the wilderness with the full knowledge that the devil will tempt him. Now, we ask God frequently to "lead us not into temptation," and in confession we always promise to avoid the "near occasions" of sin, those things that we know might tempt us.

This presents us with two challenges. The first is that we know we will experience temptation in this world and in this life. Yet we also know and promise to choose the good anyway, like Jesus does when Satan tempts him.

Most of us don't have the option of living as a hermit and living apart from the world (and even hermits experience temptation, though some might be different than the ones we experience). Instead, we're called to live in the "desert," this "vale of tears," and live in it virtuously. The other challenge is to make it a little easier on ourselves by not choosing to add temptation to our life by flirting with near occasions of sin. From now until day 40, we'll be addressing these challenges both from a spiritual and physical perspective. So, right now, as much as you might be tempted to say, "21 days was enough… let me take a little break before I jump into 40," I can't encourage you any more strongly to look at that urge and respond by planning day 22 of your workout.

DAY 22

PRAYER: The *Baltimore Catechism* points out that suffering is our biggest weapon against sin. That's right, bigger than prayer, example, or encouragement. Obviously, all suffering should be coupled with prayer, and it does provide a good example and an opportunity for encouragement. But the chief weapon against sin is suffering. And what did Jesus do in the desert? He fasted and prayed for 40 days. So that's what we're going to do.

We'll be starting something called "periodic fasting" seven days a week. "What!" you say. "Fasting every day? I'll die! Even on Good Friday and Ash Wednesday the Church says I should eat one regular meal and two smaller ones, so I'm never really that hungry! Who do you think you are? A monster? Saint Francis of Assisi?"

Wow, that was quite a diatribe. No, the Church doesn't say seven days of fasting, and, no, you won't die from what I'm proposing. Trust me a minute. I'll explain the how-to shortly, but our goal here is — in a very big way — to hear and be aware of what our basic instincts are telling us (in this instance, probably, "I'M HUNGRY! FEED ME!"), and telling them, "You don't rule me."

Fasting helps us say no to a multitude of sins that result from us just being accustomed to giving in to our base instincts: gluttony, sloth, sexual sins, intemperance, the list goes on and on. How to do it? That's part of our workout today, so let's get to it.

PERIODIC FASTING

Periodic fasting is pretty simple: don't take in calories before noon. None. You can still have your coffee, but this means no cream and no sugar in it. If you're diabetic and must have calories at certain times, fine. Then exercise self-denial in another way: abstinence from meat, or bread, or sweet things, to whatever the thing is that your body says, "Ooh yeah, that's the stuff." And obviously, if you are working graveyard shifts and asleep at noon, that's cheating. From when you wake up, don't take in calories for at least four hours. But then, and here's the other half of the equation, DO eat. Don't tell yourself: "If four hours is good, twelve hours must be better! You know what, I won't eat until next Tuesday." Eat, but eat the same size lunch you would have before. Don't double the size of the meal to compensate for fasting. Okay, that's it in a nutshell.

- **For your workout today, we're just doing 30–60 minutes of endurance heart-rate cardio, whether running, biking, swimming, hiking, etc.** Since it's your first day of periodic fasting, feel it out and discern what you can handle. For the rest of these days, it's great if you can fast in the morning, eat, and then work out a short time after that, then eat again. As you get used to it, you can still do a "fasted" workout and then eat right afterward. If your schedule requires that you work out first thing in the morning, adjust that if you can, or abstain from your "danger food group of choice" all day. Never do a workout and then continue fasting. You should always have nutrition right after a workout.

- **Plan tomorrow's workout**

DAY 23

PRAYER: You're fasting again today, obviously. We'll also start meditating on the Bible verses concerning the Temptation in Desert, and offering our fasting in union with that event in Jesus' life. Today read Matthew 4:1–2, and spend some time reflecting on it. If you're still doing the 5 minutes of silence daily, you're allowed to use that time to meditate on the verses. Otherwise, if you want to add a few extra minutes of meditation, you're encouraged to do that, too!

CROSS-TRAINING

Today's workout can be done inside or outside, if you're willing to get creative. For example, when I do this during a trail run, I'll find a tree to do my pull-ups on, or sometimes I'll run around the park and do my pull-ups on a bar at the playground. This is a flexible workout that again allows you push hard during portions, but still ease into working on an empty stomach if that's what you're doing.

- **Do a warm up jog for 5 minutes**

REPEAT THE FOLLOWING CIRCUIT 4 TIMES:
- **Run 4 minutes or 0.5 miles at a high but sustainable intensity (not sprinting pace, but not cardio endurance pace either)**

- 10 push-ups

- 5 pull-ups

- 15 crunches

- Rest only long enough to let your heart rate dip back into your endurance zone (180 minus age), then go again

- Jog 30 minutes or 3 miles

- Plan tomorrow's workout

DAY 24

PRAYER: Fast and meditate on Matthew 4:3–4.

ACTIVE RECOVERY
- Today's an easy one, because tomorrow we start a week of endurance training... so rest up and get ready!

- Plan tomorrow's workout

DAY 25

PRAYER: Fast and meditate on Matthew 4:5–7.

LEG ENDURANCE
We start training muscular endurance today, so we're going to hit legs with everything we've got.

- Warm up on the stair climber or on the highest incline treadmill for 5 minutes

TRI-SET (5 TIMES), NO REST BETWEEN EXERCISES, 1 MINUTE REST BETWEEN SETS

- **Squats, 5 sets x 40%ORM x 20 reps**

- **Romanian dead lifts, 5 sets x 50%ORM x 20 reps**

- **Squat jumps, 5 sets x 20 reps**

SUPERSET (5 TIMES), NO REST

- **1–2 minute wall sit (depending on fitness level)**

- **4-minute stair climber or highest incline on treadmill (let your heart rate come down to your endurance zone)**

- **Cool down and stretch**

- **Plan tomorrow's workout**

DAY 26

PRAYER: Fast and meditate on Matthew 4:8-10.

BACK AND BICEP ENDURANCE

- **Warm up with 5 minutes of easy rowing and stretching**

- **50 pull-ups (or inverted push-ups, if you absolutely can't do 50 pull-ups... but, again, pull-ups are the best).** Do as many as you can in a row, then rest 1 minute and go again, for as long as it takes to do 50. It may take 5 sets, it may take 10 sets, it may take 20 sets, but finish 50 pull-ups.

SUPERSET 3X

- **Alternating incline dumbbell row, 20 reps.** Each dumbbell should be about 20% of your bodyweight. You can do a little less if necessary, or a little more if possible.

- **Alternating rope pull-downs, 20 reps**

- **Rest 1 minute**

- **Barbell curl, 100 reps, try to do all 100 in a row.** If you can't, you can take 10-second rest periods when you must.

- **Reverse curl, 100 reps.** Same rule about reps and rest applies here.

- **Stretch and cool down**

DAY 27

PRAYER: Fast and meditate on Matthew 4:10–11.

CHEST, SHOULDER, AND TRICEP ENDURANCE

- **Warm up shoulders, chest, etc., with easy push-ups, shoulder circles, and stretching**

- **Bench press** (increase weight slightly each set)

- **30 reps to 90 degrees, 15 full reps, 10 pause reps, rest 1 minute**

- **25 reps to 90 degrees, 12 full reps, 8 pause reps, rest 1 minute**

- **20 reps to 90 degrees, 10 full reps, 5 pause reps, rest 1 minute**

- **15 reps to 90 degrees, 5 full reps, 3 pause reps, rest 1 minute**

- **10 reps to 90 degrees, 3 full rep, 1 pause rep, rest 1 minute**

- **Plank push-ups** (208, 209, 210, 208 again) Start in an elevated plank position, then place the left forearm on the ground, then the right, then go back to left side elevated and right side elevated. Keep alternating which side you bring down first.

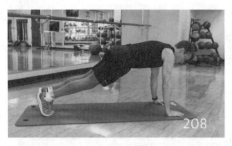

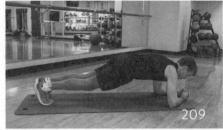

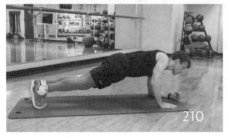

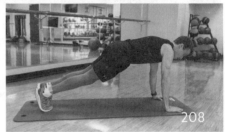

- **Super slow push-ups to failure**

- **Cable shoulder press, 100 reps** (211, 212) Place the cable pulleys low, and hold the handles at shoulder height, palms facing forward. Keeping your head and chest up, extend to press the handles directly over head. Return slowly to the starting position.

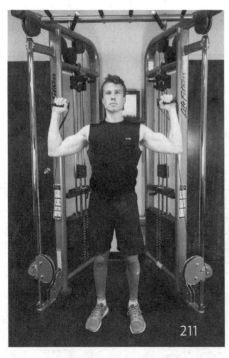

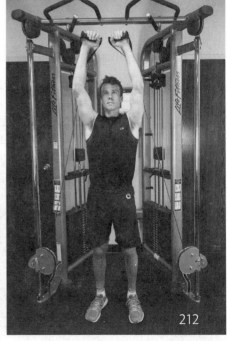

- **Rope overhead extension, 100 reps** (213, 214) Attach a rope to a low pulley and face away from the cable. Position your hands behind your head with your elbows pointing straight up, or at least close to it. Stagger your stance and lean gently away from the machine for more stability.

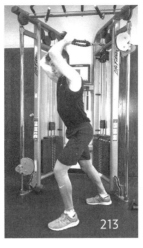 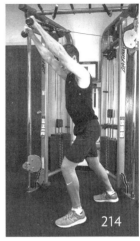

Extend your arms while keeping the upper arm still, until your arms form a straight line. Pause and return slowly to the starting position.

- **Lateral raise, 50 reps**

- **Super slow "close grip" knee push-ups to failure**

- **Stretch and cool down**

- **Plan tomorrow's workout**

DAY 28

PRAYER: Fast and meditate on Luke 4:1–2.

- **Active recovery**

- **Plan tomorrow's workout**

DAY 29

PRAYER: Fast and meditate on Luke 4:3–4.

CORE ENDURANCE

SUPERSET FOR TIME 1, 3, 5, 9, 15, 21, 15, 9, 5, 3, 1 REPS
- **Dead lift at 50% ORM** (be cautious here with your form as you get to higher reps)

- **Squat jumps**

SUPERSET X 2
- **Plank variations on a theme**

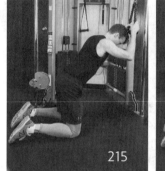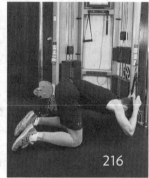

215

216

- **Ab wheel rollouts or rope crunches** (215, 216) Kneel 1–2 feet in front of a cable machine with a rope attachment on a high pulley. Hold the rope in both hands, with your torso almost upright. Flex at the spine, attempting to bring your rib cage to your legs as you pull the cable down. Pause at the bottom of the rep, and then return to the starting position.

- **Optional: Light farmer's carry** (25% bodyweight), 2 minutes on, 1 minute off, for up to 15 minutes. (217) Holding dumbbells in each hand that add up to a portion of your bodyweight (in this instance, 25%), keep your back straight, torso upright, and shoulders back, and walk either around the gym or the block, or on a treadmill.

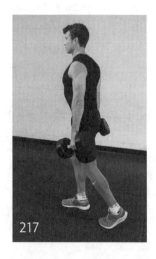

217

- **Stretch and cool down**

- **Plan tomorrow's workout**

DAY 30

PRAYER: Fast and meditate on Luke 4:5–8.

CARDIOVASCULAR ENDURANCE

A track is a great place to do this. If you don't have a public track nearby, most high schools and colleges let people from the community use their track if they have one. Check on it.

If you have an issue preventing you from running, you can do these on a bike (outside or in a gym), in a pool, on a rowing machine, etc. Basically, 30 seconds of as close to max effort as you can, followed by 2–3 minutes of active recovery, then 15–30 minutes in the cardio endurance heart-rate zone.

- Intervals, 6–12 times

- Sprint as hard as you can maintain for 30 seconds

- Jog for 2–3 minutes at a pace slow enough to recover

- Cardio endurance jog for 15–30 minutes

- Stretch and cool down

- Plan tomorrow's workout

DAY 31

PRAYER: Fast and meditate on Luke 4:9–13

- Active recovery

- Plan tomorrow's workout

DAY 32

PRAYER: Fast and meditate on Mark 1:12–13

- **Active recovery** (What? 2 days of active recovery in a row? Yep. Last week was tough! Give yourself a pat on the back!)

- **Plan tomorrow's workout** (which won't be active recovery)

DAY 33

PRAYER: Fast and meditate on Matthew 4:1–4

BODYWEIGHT PULL DAY

We're doing a bodyweight-only workout week. If you love it, continue to incorporate it — or elements like it — regularly, particularly if you're training for something like an obstacle race. If you don't love it, or you hate it, okay, you don't have to do it again after this week. But doing bodyweight exercises makes sure that you're going through movements that your body is made to do, rather than some movements that are more isolated. We're pulling a lot today, so find a park or place that has at least one horizontal bar you can do pull-ups on and one vertical bar you can do rows on.

TRI-SET 3X
- **Pull-ups, 5–10 reps**

- **Crunches, 20 reps**

- **Bicycles, 20 reps (10 each side)** (218, 219) Lying on your back with your legs slightly elevated and your shoulders just off the ground, keep your abs tight and alternate bringing your opposite elbow to knee. Keep your legs elevated and core tight through the exercise.

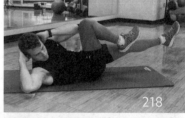
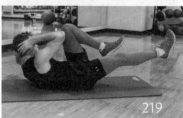

SUPERSET 3X

- Towel rows, 10–15 reps

- Mountain climbers, 20 reps (10 each side)

- Plank, 30 seconds — 1 minute

- Jog, bike, swim, trail run at an easy pace for 15 minutes — 1 hour

- Plan tomorrow's workout

DAY 34

PRAYER: Fast and meditate on Matthew 4:5–7

BODYWEIGHT PUSH DAY

- **Burpees, 30 reps.** Knock 'em out, whether it takes you 2 minutes or 10.

- Rest 1–2 minutes max

TRI-SET 3X

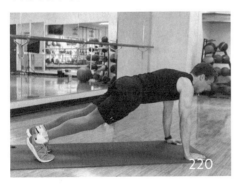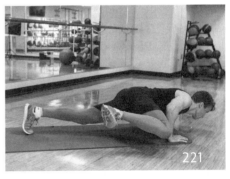

- **Spiderman push-ups or 8-count bodybuilders, 5–10 reps** (220, 221) Perform a regular push-up, but as you bring your body down, bring one knee forward to almost touch your elbow. Return to the first position, then switch sides. (222, 223, 224, 225, 226, 227, 228, 229, 230) 8-count bodybuilders take you through eight positions. Do them cleanly. 1. Squat until you can place your hands on the ground. 2. Jump back to a push-up

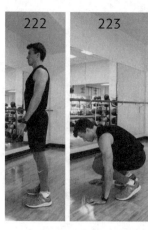
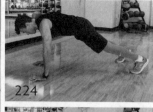
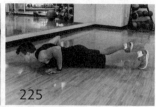
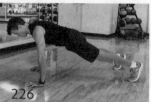
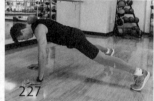
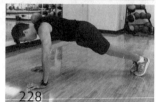

position. 3. Lower your body to the ground. 4. Push up back to push-up position. 5. Jump slightly to split your legs. 6. Jump slightly to bring your legs back together. 7. Jump back to a squatting position. 8. Stand back up

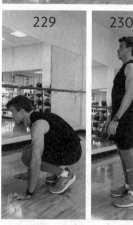

- **Bear crawl 1 minute** (231, 232, 233) Start with a body angle anywhere between a triangle (which emphasizes shoulders more) and a flat push-up position (which emphasizes core more), keeping your back flat no matter which position you choose. With hands shoulder width apart, move the left hand and the right leg forward to start crawling. Alternate arm and leg movements while keeping the back straight.

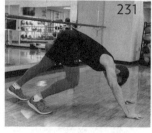
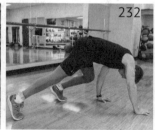
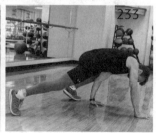

- **Crunches, 20 reps**

SUPERSET 2X

- **Super-slow push-ups to failure**

- **Bicycles, 20 reps** (10 each side)

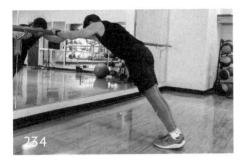
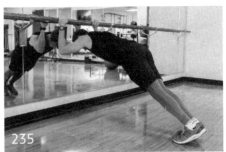

- **Tricep overhead extension for 15 reps on low bar, if you have one.** (234, 235) Find a low bar and support yourself on it with straight arms, forming as close to a straight line with your arms and body as you can. Bend your elbows and lean your body forward, dipping beneath the bar, until your forearm and upper arm form slightly less than a 90-degree angle. Push up and back with your triceps to return to the starting position. Otherwise narrow-grip knee push-ups to failure.

- **Rest 1 minute**

- **Jog, bike, swim, trail run at an easy pace for 15 minutes — 1 hour**

- **Cool down and stretch**

- **Plan tomorrow's workout**

DAY 35

PRAYER: Fast and meditate on Matthew 4:8–10

- **Active recovery**

- **Plan tomorrow's workout**

DAY 36

PRAYER: Fast and meditate on Matthew 4:10–11

BODYWEIGHT LEGS DAY

- **Squats, 100 reps.** There's no weight here except your body, so power through, and get to 100 reps. Pause if you need to, for 15 seconds max, then get back to it.

- **Rest 1 minute**

TRI-SET 3X

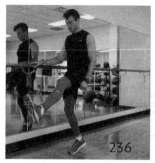 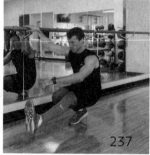 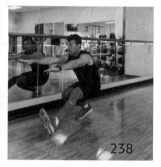

236   237   238

- **Pistol squats, 1–5 reps each side.** (236, 237, 238) From a standing position, extend one leg in front of you as you look forward, chest up, back straight. Descend into a squat, keeping your non-working leg forward and off the ground, and your knees behind your toes. Go as far down as flexibility and strength allow, then return to the starting position by extending from the hips and knee, driving down with the heel of your working foot. If necessary, you can place a hand on a bar or bench for balance. Do not use that arm to pull yourself up.

- **Crunches, 20 reps**

- **Sprint 20 seconds**

- **Rest 1 minute**

- **Jog, bike, swim, trail run at an easy pace for 15 minutes — 1 hour**

- Cool down and stretch

- Plan tomorrow's workout

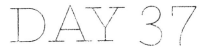
DAY 37

PRAYER: Fast and meditate on Luke 4:1–2

- Active recovery

- Plan tomorrow's workout

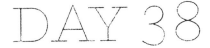
DAY 38

PRAYER: Fast and meditate on Luke 4:3–4

THE LONG RUN
- **Run 45–90 minutes, or other cardiovascular exercise in your endurance heart-rate zone**

- **Plan tomorrow's workout**

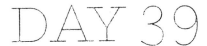
DAY 39

PRAYER: Fast and meditate on Luke 4:5–8

BODYWEIGHT FULL BODY DAY
- **Quad set, 8 times (reps listed by exercise).** Your reps are different by exercise, so the first time through, do 15 pull-ups followed by 30 push-ups, 30 crunches, 30 seconds of hard running, then start the next set.

- Pull-ups (or towel rows if you absolutely must, but I'd rather have you fight through reps) 15, 13, 11, 9, 7, 5, 3, 1

- Push-ups (knee push-ups if you must) 30, 26, 22, 18, 14, 10, 6, 2

- Crunches (legs elevated for an extra challenge) 30, 26, 22, 18, 14, 10, 6, 2

- Run hard 30 seconds, 30, 25, 25, 20, 20, 15, 15

- Rest max 30 seconds

- Cool down and stretch

- Plan tomorrow's workout

DAY 40

PRAYER: Fast and meditate on Luke 4:9–13

- Active recovery

- Plan tomorrow's workout

90 DAYS TO CHANGE YOUR LIFE

There's an adage in the world of fitness that goes like this: in 90 days (or 12 weeks, or 3 months) you can train your body to do just about anything. Well, anything within reason. Going from totally sedentary to winning a marathon may not be realistic. But walking a marathon might be. Going from not being able to do one push-up to bench pressing a small car may not be realistic. But benching your bodyweight might be. Basically, every 90 days you can make a quantum leap in your fitness.

To give you an example, five years ago, I had basically gone a full year without working out or eating right. I had a background of training, but I had left it behind. I decided to change that, and started training to do an obstacle race. Just 12 weeks later, I finished my first Spartan Race: 4 miles of running (prior to that training, I hadn't run at all in six years), 1,000 feet of elevation gain, and 20 obstacles. And 12 weeks after that, I had my old strength back in the gym. And 12 weeks after that I completed a 12-mile, 2,500-foot elevation gain, 40-obstacle race in 110-degree heat. The point isn't to brag, but to demonstrate that from where I started to where I ended in each 12-week period really was a completely different level of fitness.

To give another example, my brother was more than 20 pounds overweight, and he decided he wanted to make a change. In three months, he lost 22 pounds (and a month later had dropped another 8), just through dedicating himself to eating a calorie-restricted diet and cycling regularly. A couple years later, he decided he wanted to add muscle and gained 15 pounds of it in a 12-week period by working out regularly and eating appropriately for his goals. He's a very focused dude, and this shows what's possible if you are willing to be focused.

It all comes down to ownership. If you're willing to hone in on what your goals are, get specific, be accountable, and follow through, with a little faith, you will move mountains. This holds true for both body and soul. You cannot possibly avoid being changed for good if you start and end each day with gratitude to God and spend at least five minutes a day in silence with him. If you eat and train properly for your goals, you cannot possibly avoid being changed. As always, the key is to do it — and keep doing it.

If, on the other hand, when you see change you begin to rest on your laurels, or look at it as an occasion for pride instead of gratitude, you'll end up like the man in the parable of the seven demons from Matthew 12:43–45:

> "When the unclean spirit has gone out of a man, he passes through waterless places seeking rest, but he finds none. Then he says, 'I will return to my house from which I came.' And when he comes he finds it empty, swept, and put in order. Then he goes and brings with him seven other spirits more evil than himself, and they enter and dwell there; and the last state of that man becomes worse than the first."

You see this all the time in athletes who stop playing their sport, or in people who dive deeply into their faith for a time but get "burnt out." They neglect daily practice, gratitude, and humility, and end up out of shape physically or spiritually, and become a scandal to others. Don't do that.

With ownership, accountability, and focus in mind, here comes your big 90-day challenge: you create a workout plan, for body and soul. "*What!*" you ask, "Wait a minute, I bought this book because it said it had a 9-, 21-, 40-, and 90-day workout plan!" Well, it does... it has the best 90-day workout plan possible, because it's a workout plan designed specifically for *you* and *your* goals.

Don't worry, I'm not leaving you high and dry here. We're about to break down how to craft it, and we have space for you to write it all in. But every 90 days from here until the end of your life can serve as a great period to reevaluate where you are, where you're going, and if you're really on the track to get there. If you're not, no problem. Just figure out what you need to do to change course and get back on track.

We've explored gratitude, stillness and silent prayer, virtue and habits, temptation and meditation. We've looked at exercises to build strength, speed, endurance, and flexibility. You now have dozens at your disposal. So let's start building the right path for the 90 days that will change your life!

What Are Your Goals?

Goals serve as the starting point for any plan. G. K. Chesterton says: "Progress should mean that we are always changing the world to suit the vision. Progress does mean (just now) that we are always changing the vision." There's no such thing as progress unless you have a specific idea of where you actually want to get to, what you want to change, and what you want to change it to.

What do you want to change in your life? Pick a spiritual goal and a physical goal. Here are some jumping-off points do get you thinking:

SPIRITUAL GOALS
- Make a daily practice of prayer or meditation
- Grow in intimacy with God
- Open myself more to the Holy Spirit
- Learn more about my faith
- Do more for others
- Let the graces God has given me lead and inform my life more
- Receive a sacrament five days a week
- Shut off my phone after 10 p.m. and fast from social media
- Do the Spiritual Exercises of Saint Ignatius

PHYSICAL GOALS
- Drop my body fat percentage three points
- Finish a race (5k, obstacle race, cycle, swim, marathon, cross-country ski)
- Gain 5–10 pounds of muscle
- Increase strength by 10–20%
- Run, swim, or cycle a specific distance
- Work out 5 days a week for 12 weeks
- Meet all the flexibility standards while developing corresponding strength

What Is Your Plan?

Every day for the last 40 days, I've had you plan the next day's workout. Today, I'd encourage you to both figure out what the next 50 days look like as a whole, generally speaking, and to lay out your next week of workouts (both spiritual and physical) specifically. If you want to develop strength, what exercises, rest, and nutrition will get you there? How about if you want to lose fat? What about training for a race? How will you plug in the components of fitness and the exercises you've learned to get you where you'd like to be?

On the spiritual side, how will you grow in the next 50 days? If it's self-discipline you're after, what daily practice will make that feasible? What does growing in intimacy with God look like? Do you need to make more time for prayer and the sacraments, or less space for distractions and near occasions of sin? And in all of it, how do *ora et labora* (prayer and work) come together? How will you let the physical and the spiritual be integrated as one instead of separate parts? Write out a week, and set goals for yourself over the course of the next 50 days.

How Will You Continue to Learn?

In looking at your goals, you may already realize you want and need more knowledge to get there. The first piece of advice I would give you is get started *today*. Don't put it off one more day or one more minute just because "I need to know more." You'll always have more to learn. Start the journey anyway, and find guidebooks along the way. Always be learning, always be growing, always be changing. Every day my friend Joseph Pearce spends one hour praying, one hour reading, and one hour training so that he's dedicating an hour a day each to soul, mind, and body. While that may not be entirely possible for everyone, I think that it's an awesome protocol to work from.

Now, if in looking at your goals for the next 50 days you think you have sufficient knowledge to accomplish them, great! You can already start learning for the next 12 weeks. Remember whatever goal or goals took second place when you were deciding what you wanted to do. Spend time learning about those, so you can jump into them once these 90 days are up. But either way, at the end of 90 days be sure to have your goals lined up for the next 90 days, lest you "invite seven demons" back in the place of the one you've driven out!

How Will You Stay Accountable?

The final key to growing — as you might remember from early in this book — is to have relationships that keep you accountable and on the right path. To again refer to Ecclesiastes 4:12: "And though a man might prevail against one who is alone, two will withstand him. A threefold cord is not quickly broken."

I can't tell you how many times my training partners have clued me in to something new they were learning, which helped me take my training, my dieting, or my recovery to the next level. The same holds true with a good spiritual director and friends walking the walk of faith — people who've seen where I'm at, observed my strengths and struggles, and can provide insight, encouragement, and empathy.

While I specifically challenged you to join a gym early on in your workouts, and then to use the gym, I didn't require you to get a training partner. If you've managed to make it to day 40 without a training partner, day 41 is where you get one. Seriously.

Within the next 24 hours, get a "workout date" (not like a romantic date, just, you know, a training date) on the calendar with someone, and make sure it's within the next week. Actually, better yet, get two workout dates on the schedule, in case your first attempt at a training partner no-shows or something (because you certainly won't be the one no-showing… right?). After you've done that, or if you are already working with a training partner, share your goals with them so they can provide the support you need and the help you want. Then, offer the same assistance to them in return. This also applies for spiritual training partners (and if you find a person who can be one and the same, great!). That person needs to know where you're coming from and where you're going to if they're going to be a helpmate to you.

All right, that's it. I hope I've been a help to you. In John 14:12, Jesus said, "Truly, truly, I say to you, he who believes in me will also do the works that I do; and greater works than these will he do." Jesus also tells us that with faith the size of a mustard seed, we will move mountains (see Mt 17:20).

So… in your faith — in your whole wonderful, integrated life of body and soul and heart and mind — let nothing be impossible with God, be not afraid, and do great works for the greater glory of God.

Amen.

DAY 41

PRAYER: _____

_____

_____

_____

_____

_____

WORKOUT: _____

_____

_____

_____

_____

_____

_____

_____

_____

_____

_____

_____

DAY 42

PRAYER: _____

_____

_____

_____

_____

_____

_____

WORKOUT: _____

_____

_____

_____

_____

_____

_____

_____

_____

_____

_____

_____

_____

_____

DAY 43

PRAYER: _____

_____

_____

_____

_____

_____

WORKOUT: _____

_____

_____

_____

_____

_____

_____

_____

_____

_____

_____

_____

_____

DAY 44

PRAYER: _____

_____

_____

_____

_____

_____

_____

WORKOUT: _____

_____

_____

_____

_____

_____

_____

_____

_____

_____

_____

_____

_____

DAY 45

PRAYER: _____

_____

_____

_____

_____

_____

_____

WORKOUT: _____

_____

_____

_____

_____

_____

_____

_____

_____

_____

_____

_____

_____

_____

DAY 46

PRAYER: _____

_____

_____

_____

_____

_____

_____

WORKOUT: _____

_____

_____

_____

_____

_____

_____

_____

_____

_____

_____

_____

_____

_____

DAY 47

PRAYER: _____

_____

_____

_____

_____

_____

WORKOUT: _____

_____

_____

_____

_____

_____

_____

_____

_____

_____

_____

_____

_____

DAY 48

PRAYER: _____

_____

_____

_____

_____

_____

WORKOUT: _____

_____

_____

_____

_____

_____

_____

_____

_____

_____

_____

_____

_____

DAY 49

PRAYER: _____

_____

_____

_____

_____

_____

WORKOUT: _____

_____

_____

_____

_____

_____

_____

_____

_____

_____

_____

_____

_____

DAY 50

PRAYER: _____

_____

_____

_____

_____

_____

WORKOUT: _____

_____

_____

_____

_____

_____

_____

_____

_____

_____

_____

_____

_____

DAY 51

PRAYER: _____

_____

_____

_____

_____

_____

WORKOUT: _____

_____

_____

_____

_____

_____

_____

_____

_____

_____

_____

_____

_____

DAY 52

PRAYER: _____

_____

_____

_____

_____

_____

_____

WORKOUT: _____

_____

_____

_____

_____

_____

_____

_____

_____

_____

_____

_____

_____

DAY 53

PRAYER: _____

_____

_____

_____

_____

_____

WORKOUT: _____

_____

_____

_____

_____

_____

_____

_____

_____

_____

_____

_____

_____

DAY 54

PRAYER: _____

_____

_____

_____

_____

_____

WORKOUT: _____

_____

_____

_____

_____

_____

_____

_____

_____

_____

_____

_____

_____

DAY 55

PRAYER: _____

_____

_____

_____

_____

_____

WORKOUT: _____

_____

_____

_____

_____

_____

_____

_____

_____

_____

_____

_____

_____

DAY 56

PRAYER: _____

_____

_____

_____

_____

_____

WORKOUT: _____

_____

_____

_____

_____

_____

_____

_____

_____

_____

_____

_____

DAY 57

PRAYER: _____

_____

_____

_____

_____

_____

WORKOUT: _____

_____

_____

_____

_____

_____

_____

_____

_____

_____

_____

_____

DAY 58

PRAYER: _____

_____

_____

_____

_____

_____

WORKOUT: _____

_____

_____

_____

_____

_____

_____

_____

_____

_____

_____

_____

DAY 59

PRAYER: _____

_____

_____

_____

_____

_____

WORKOUT: _____

_____

_____

_____

_____

_____

_____

_____

_____

_____

_____

_____

_____

DAY 60

PRAYER: _____

_____

_____

_____

_____

_____

_____

WORKOUT: _____

_____

_____

_____

_____

_____

_____

_____

_____

_____

_____

_____

_____

DAY 61

PRAYER: _____

_____

_____

_____

_____

_____

WORKOUT: _____

_____

_____

_____

_____

_____

_____

_____

_____

_____

_____

_____

_____

DAY 62

PRAYER: _____

_____

_____

_____

_____

_____

_____

WORKOUT: _____

_____

_____

_____

_____

_____

_____

_____

_____

_____

_____

_____

DAY 63

PRAYER: _____

_____

_____

_____

_____

_____

WORKOUT: _____

_____

_____

_____

_____

_____

_____

_____

_____

_____

_____

_____

_____

DAY 64

PRAYER: _____

_____

_____

_____

_____

_____

_____

WORKOUT: _____

_____

_____

_____

_____

_____

_____

_____

_____

_____

_____

_____

_____

_____

DAY 65

PRAYER: _____

_____

_____

_____

_____

_____

_____

WORKOUT: _____

_____

_____

_____

_____

_____

_____

_____

_____

_____

_____

_____

_____

_____

_____

DAY 66

PRAYER: _____

_____

_____

_____

_____

_____

WORKOUT: _____

_____

_____

_____

_____

_____

_____

_____

_____

_____

_____

_____

_____

DAY 67

PRAYER: _____

_____

_____

_____

_____

_____

_____

WORKOUT: _____

_____

_____

_____

_____

_____

_____

_____

_____

_____

_____

_____

_____

_____

_____

DAY 68

PRAYER: _____

_____

_____

_____

_____

_____

_____

WORKOUT: _____

_____

_____

_____

_____

_____

_____

_____

_____

_____

_____

_____

_____

DAY 69

PRAYER: _____

_____

_____

_____

_____

_____

WORKOUT: _____

_____

_____

_____

_____

_____

_____

_____

_____

_____

_____

_____

_____

DAY 70

PRAYER: _____

_____

_____

_____

_____

_____

WORKOUT: _____

_____

_____

_____

_____

_____

_____

_____

_____

_____

_____

_____

DAY 71

PRAYER: _____

_____

_____

_____

_____

_____

_____

WORKOUT: _____

_____

_____

_____

_____

_____

_____

_____

_____

_____

_____

_____

_____

_____

DAY 72

PRAYER:

_____

_____

_____

_____

_____

_____

WORKOUT:

_____

_____

_____

_____

_____

_____

_____

_____

_____

_____

_____

_____

DAY 73

PRAYER: _____

_____

_____

_____

_____

_____

WORKOUT: _____

_____

_____

_____

_____

_____

_____

_____

_____

_____

_____

_____

_____

DAY 74

PRAYER: _____

_____

_____

_____

_____

_____

WORKOUT: _____

_____

_____

_____

_____

_____

_____

_____

_____

_____

_____

_____

DAY 75

PRAYER: _____

_____

_____

_____

_____

_____

WORKOUT: _____

_____

_____

_____

_____

_____

_____

_____

_____

_____

_____

_____

_____

_____

DAY 76

PRAYER: _____

_____

_____

_____

_____

_____

WORKOUT: _____

_____

_____

_____

_____

_____

_____

_____

_____

_____

_____

_____

_____

DAY 77

PRAYER: _____

_____

_____

_____

_____

_____

WORKOUT: _____

_____

_____

_____

_____

_____

_____

_____

_____

_____

_____

_____

_____

DAY 78

PRAYER: _____

_____

_____

_____

_____

_____

_____

WORKOUT: _____

_____

_____

_____

_____

_____

_____

_____

_____

_____

_____

_____

_____

DAY 79

PRAYER: _____

_____

_____

_____

_____

_____

WORKOUT: _____

_____

_____

_____

_____

_____

_____

_____

_____

_____

_____

_____

DAY 80

PRAYER:

_____

_____

_____

_____

_____

_____

_____

WORKOUT:

_____

_____

_____

_____

_____

_____

_____

_____

_____

_____

_____

_____

_____

DAY 81

PRAYER: _____

_____

_____

_____

_____

_____

_____

WORKOUT: _____

_____

_____

_____

_____

_____

_____

_____

_____

_____

_____

_____

_____

DAY 82

PRAYER: _____

_____

_____

_____

_____

_____

_____

WORKOUT: _____

_____

_____

_____

_____

_____

_____

_____

_____

_____

_____

_____

_____

DAY 83

PRAYER: _____

_____

_____

_____

_____

_____

WORKOUT: _____

_____

_____

_____

_____

_____

_____

_____

_____

_____

_____

_____

DAY 84

PRAYER: _____

_____

_____

_____

_____

_____

WORKOUT: _____

_____

_____

_____

_____

_____

_____

_____

_____

_____

_____

_____

DAY 85

PRAYER: _____

_____

_____

_____

_____

_____

_____

WORKOUT: _____

_____

_____

_____

_____

_____

_____

_____

_____

_____

_____

_____

_____

_____

DAY 86

PRAYER: _____

_____

_____

_____

_____

_____

WORKOUT: _____

_____

_____

_____

_____

_____

_____

_____

_____

_____

_____

_____

DAY 87

PRAYER: _____

_____

_____

_____

_____

_____

WORKOUT: _____

_____

_____

_____

_____

_____

_____

_____

_____

_____

_____

_____

DAY 88

PRAYER: _____

_____

_____

_____

_____

_____

WORKOUT: _____

_____

_____

_____

_____

_____

_____

_____

_____

_____

_____

_____

_____

DAY 89

PRAYER: _____

_____

_____

_____

_____

_____

WORKOUT: _____

_____

_____

_____

_____

_____

_____

_____

_____

_____

_____

_____

DAY 90

PRAYER: _____

_____

_____

_____

_____

_____

WORKOUT: _____

_____

_____

_____

_____

_____

_____

_____

_____

_____

_____

_____

_____

STRETCHES SUPPLEMENT

Quad stretch (239) Stand upright on one leg, bring your other leg up behind you, with the upper legs parallel, and try to bring your heel to touch your butt.

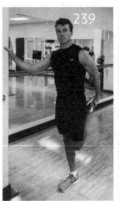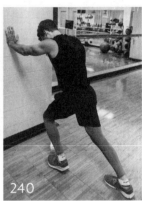

Calf stretch (240) Stand in a lunged position, pushing against a wall, with the rear leg at a 45-degree angle to the wall. Try to bring the heel of the rear leg to the ground, then lean further into the stretch.

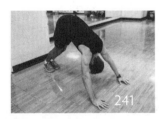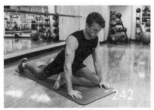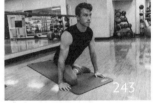

Pigeon stretch for hips and legs (241, 242, 243) From a pike position, swing one leg up and bring it forward, in between your hands, and place it at as close to a 90-degree angle as you can. Keep your back leg straight behind you, and try to continue to bring your butt closer to the ground and your front leg closer to 90 degrees.

Cobra stretch for core (244) From lying flat on the ground with your hands in a push-up position, straighten your arms. To vary the stretch, you can either keep your hips on the ground or slightly elevate them.

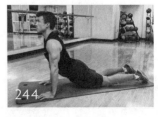

Extended reach for back, hips, and legs (245) Sit back on your heels and extend your arms in front of you. Keep your back flat or slightly rounded and your neck relaxed.

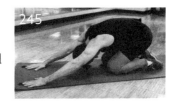

Egg-crackers (246, 247) Roll back gently so your legs come back over your head, then roll forward so you come to a seated and reaching position. Repeat.

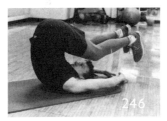
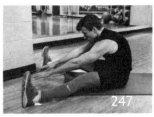

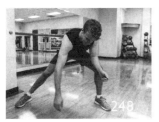
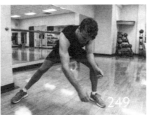
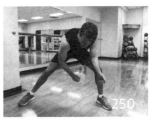

Pot-stirrers for back (248, 249, 250) Leaning against one leg, relax your arm and swing it in a circle several times. Reverse direction. Repeat for the other arm.

Static back stretch (251, 252) Holding onto a low bar (either vertical or horizontal), gently push hips backward to feel a stretch along your back muscle. Switch sides.

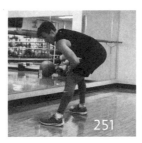
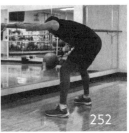

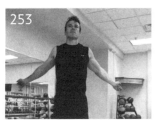
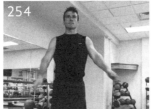
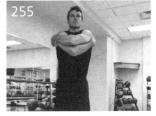

Hug stretch for chest (253, 254, 255) Swing your arms back and forth between a hugging position and outstretched (as far as is comfortable).

Static chest and arm stretch (256, 257) Stretch one arm to your side against a wall, then rotate your body so your arm starts to move behind you (as far as is comfortable, up to just past perpendicular). Keep your hand flat to stretch your chest, turn it sideways to stretch your biceps.

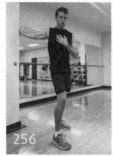 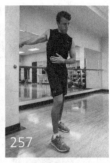

Static overhead tricep stretch (258, 259) Bend one arm back at the elbow over the shoulder, as if trying to do the back-scratch test. Gently push that elbow further in line with your body using your other hand.

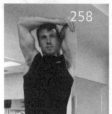 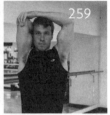

Static forearm stretch (260, 261) Gently pull your hand until your wrist is a 90-degree angle, then push your hand forward until your wrist is a 90-degree angle the other direction.

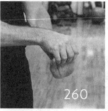 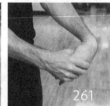

Static shoulder stretch (262) Pull one relaxed arm across your body using the other arm just above the upper arm from the elbow.

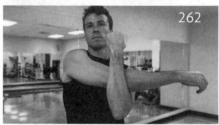

Static behind-the-back neck stretch (263, 264) Place one hand behind your back and gently pull it using your other arm. Gently lean your head the same direction you're pulling your arm.

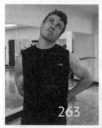 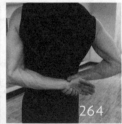

Static neck turns (265) Turn your head to one side and apply very gentle pressure to your chin to hold the stretch.

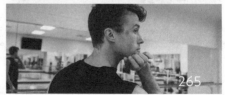